Praise for *Bea* *Brazilian Beau*

"A unique work of art. E ~~~ attest to its unparalleled contribution to the genre... It offers an elegant and intelligent holistic approach to good health and happiness the Brazilian way... and the world has definitely witnessed this power in past decades. This book is a must-read!"
  —**Anne Devi Wold, MD, Brown University Assistant Clinical Professor and Yale University Clinical Instructor of Gynecology and Women's Health**

"*Beauty Is Power: Dr. Luciano's Brazilian Beauty Secrets for Staying Young* is a must-read for everyone concerned about outer and inner beauty... Truly inspirational."
  —**Shanna Moakler, Miss USA 1995**

"A health and beauty prescription for success... A sound mind in a sound body... A very positive approach."
  —**Alon J. Vainer, MD, FACP, Clinical Assistant Professor of Medicine, Medical College of Georgia**

"A remarkable and inspirational book... Its principles, revelations, and insights will be cherished by men and women."
  —**Dr. Jeff Newman, Health Source of Providence, Rhode Island**

"An inspirational, lifestyle-affirming creation. Dr. Luciano blends science with the proven track record of a culture where beauty is nurtured as a fundamental right."
  —**Marshall Wold, MD, Psychiatrist, East Bay Center, Rhode Island**

"Nobody knows beauty—or Brazil—better than Dr. Luciano, and he has put all his knowledge together in a concise, brilliant style... This book is a powerful guide for anyone looking to improve their looks and health—and who isn't?"
  —**M.C. Ghefter, MD, Chief of Thoracic Surgery, HSPE Hospital, São Paulo, Brazil**

BEAUTY IS POWER

Dr. Luciano's Brazilian Beauty Secrets for Staying Young

BEAUTY IS POWER

Dr. Luciano's Brazilian Beauty Secrets for Staying Young

Luciano Sztulman, MD, FACS, FACOG

ARIMEL ENTERPRISES

Beauty Is Power:
Dr. Luciano's Brazilian Beauty Secrets for Staying Young
Copyright © 2013 Luciano Sztulman, MD, FACS, FACOG
Published by Arimel Enterprises

All rights reserved. No part of this book may be reproduced (except for inclusion in reviews), disseminated or utilized in any form or by any means, electronic or mechanical, including photocopying, recording, or in any information storage and retrieval system, or the Internet/World Wide Web without written permission from the author or publisher.

For more information contact:
Luciano Sztulman, MD
One Randall Square, Suite 401
Providence, RI 02904
E-mail: doc@beautyispower.us

Printed in the United States of America

Beauty Is Power:
Dr. Luciano's Brazilian Beauty Secrets for Staying Young
Luciano Sztulman, MD, FACS, FACOG

1. Title   2. Author   3. Health/Beauty

Library of Congress Control Number: 2012918772

ISBN 13: 978-0-615-70885-0

TABLE OF CONTENTS

ACKNOWLEDGMENTS xi

SECTION I
Brazilian Wonder

CHAPTER 1
Brazil's Long History of Beauty and Youthfulness 3

CHAPTER 2
Natural Botanicals and Science:
The Modern-Day Fountains of Youth 11

SECTION II
We Are What We Eat—Brazilian Diet Secrets

CHAPTER 3
The Crippling Effect: Foods That Make You Age 21

CHAPTER 4
The Brazilian Bounty: Natural Foods for Youthfulness 29

CHAPTER 5
Bridging the Brazilian Gap: Nutritional Supplements........... 37

CHAPTER 6
Brazilian Cleansing:
Detoxification and Dietary Toxin Avoidance........................... 45

SECTION III
We Are How We Live—The Brazilian Lifestyle

CHAPTER 7
The Energy of Brazil: A Passion for Exercise and Fitness 55

CHAPTER 8
The Brazilian Work Ethic: Staying Mentally Active 61

CHAPTER 9
Brazilian Balance:
Making Time for Sleep and Relaxation 69

CHAPTER 10
The Brazilian Body: One Size Does Not Fit All 77

CHAPTER 11
The Nature of Brazil: Avoiding Environmental Toxins 83

SECTION IV
We Are How We Feel: The Brazilian Philosophy

CHAPTER 12
An Expressive People: Brazil's Secret to Emotional Health ... 93

CHAPTER 13
Brazil's Formula for Stress:
Family, Friends, and Forever Young 101

CHAPTER 14
Spirituality and Youth: The Soul of Brazil 107

CHAPTER 15
Desire for Beauty: Is It All about Sex? 115

SECTION V
We Are How We Look: The Brazilian Insight

CHAPTER 16
Brazilian Cleanliness: Health and Hygiene 125

CHAPTER 17
Brazil's Ancient Secret: Natural Skin Care Strategies 131

CHAPTER 18
International Trendsetters:
Brazilian Beauty in Fashion and Style 137

CHAPTER 19
The Brazilian Approach:
Plastic Versus Nonplastic Interventions 143

SECTION VI
A Prescription for Youth, Brazilian Style

CHAPTER 20
Adopting a Brazilian Attitude 151

CHAPTER 21
Youth-Promoting Brazilian Recipes 159

CHAPTER 22
Brazilian Passion for Fitness 167

CHAPTER 23
Skin Products with Some of Brazil's Best-Kept Secrets 175

CHAPTER 24
Beauty Is Power: Brazil's Fountain of Youth 183

AUTHOR'S NOTE 189

ENDNOTES 193

INDEX 207

NOTES 209

ABOUT THE AUTHOR 211

ACKNOWLEDGMENTS

I dedicate this book to my wife, planner, organizer, and right hand, Karen; and to my daughters, Arielle and Melanie. Thank you all for the love and support, and for making me such a happy husband and father.

Many relatives, friends, and coworkers contributed to this book in many different ways, both directly and indirectly. I consider myself privileged to have had such unique opportunities, and I would like to thank you all very much for your support.

Thanks to my sisters, Miriam, Gisela, and Noemi.

Thanks to Paulo Schenberg, Oswaldo and Claudio Berbel, and Ana Flavia Perel.

A very special thanks to my parents, David and Menucha Sztulman, for the love, education and support over the years. How I wish you were here!

Thanks to Mario, Jose, and Dorita Ghefter; Liliana Seger Jacob; Moshe Laufer; Edilberto Luciano Mendes; and all my patients for their trust and confidence.

—Luciano Sztulman, MD

SECTION I
Brazilian Wonder

CHAPTER 1

Brazil's Long History of Beauty and Youthfulness

Imagine lying on Rio de Janeiro's sun-soaked sands, surrounded by its stunning blue waters while sipping refreshing coconut water. In the background plays a familiar but forgotten song, "The Girl from Ipanema," and you immerse yourself in the elegance, beauty, and agelessness of the moment. Amidst the hypnotic, sensual rhythms and glistening, tan bodies, you realize this place has been forgotten by time. Somehow, this nirvana has escaped what has been assumed to be the inevitable. Magnificence and splendor abound, and you absorb every ounce possible, fearing it may soon evaporate into thin air. But this is Brazil, the land of youth and beauty. And with it comes Brazil's true secret of success: personal empowerment.

When we first hear the phrase "beauty is power," our own culture has taught us this statement is a myth. After all, beauty is supposedly skin deep. Immediately the assumption is the beauty described refers to outer beauty at the expense of inner elegance. But why must we distinguish between the two? Research has demonstrated that the lack of a positive attitude is associated with an inability to flourish.[1] Likewise, poor health habits affecting our inner body soon become evident on the outside as well.[2] In contrast, we all can appreciate the feelings enjoyed when we are fashionably dressed, physically attractive, and sexually appealing. These are just as much ingredients of empowerment as are spirituality, optimism, and inner courage. Brazilians have long realized this as an important ingredient to human success.

Brazil—Unique Culture Dedicated to Youth and Beauty

Brazil's reputation for sensuality, beauty, and youthfulness originates within multicultural influences. Despite the Portuguese initially discovering and colonizing Brazil since 1500, an influx of Dutch, Italian, German, and Spanish immigrants populated many areas of the country in centuries to follow. Likewise, the demands for harvesting brazilwood and sugarcane prompted the use of African slaves, which also influenced the national culture.[3] The end result has been a unique brand of cuisine, fashion, expression, and lifestyle that has nurtured Brazilians to perceive all forms of beauty as empowering. As a result, the Brazilian fusion of inner and outer beauty has created international awareness of its culture in respect not only to antiaging secrets but also to health in general.

One of the most notable aspects of Brazilian culture is dance. The samba, which has been a part of Brazilian culture since the late nineteenth century, reflects a blend of African and Portuguese cultures and presents a provocative and exhilarating movement of the body.[4] While as much as 400 calories may be burned in an hour of samba dancing, the actual expression and sensuality of the dance is equally important to youthfulness and health. The samba, as well as its later counterpart, the bossa nova, reflects the openness of the Brazilian people to other cultures and new ideas. Such behaviors have been linked to positive health.[5] The vibrancy and energy associated with such Brazilian dances have long been perceived as not only stunning but also as a means to perpetual youthfulness in body, mind, and spirit.

In my own experience, having spent my childhood and young adulthood in São Paulo, this vibrancy among Brazilians is exemplified in every aspect of their lifestyle. My parents and I, along with many others, suffered many hardships during the inflationary years of the 1970s through the 1990s. Suddenly we found ourselves as part of the lower middle class and struggling to make ends meet. But Brazilians retain hope and adapt easily to challenges, both of which have been associated with health and youthfulness.[6] In Brazil, a smart man is not only the one who received a special diploma or degree but also one dedicated to his family and able to survive while making minimum wage. The importance of mental adaptability runs deep within Brazilian culture and fosters a positive attitude, vitality, and youth in a large way.

Embracing their typical strong work ethic while looking for new ways to excel, Brazilians have repeatedly bounced back from struggles with a passion. In fact, passion and warmth lie within the heart of every Brazilian. In everything they do, Brazilians thoroughly invest themselves toward a goal and do so with powerful optimism and energy. With intensity and passion, their focus remains on the positive and never the negative, which is why over and over again Brazil has surprised the world with its achievements. As has been their course through history, Brazilians manifest their own destiny by infusing their lifestyle and culture with invigorating passion.

Even when times were tough, Brazilians remained dedicated to beauty. Appearance is as important as language, body movement, and behavior in Brazil. Whether wearing a small piece of fabric at the beach or dressed in an elaborate Carnival costume, Brazilians pay great attention to the fashion and trends of the day. In a way, such dedication is a means by which empowerment can persist even in the face of challenge. Beauty and youth thus form necessary ingredients for resiliency when the going gets tough. In support of this philosophy, and budget permitting, many Brazilians change their wardrobes several times a year to stay trendy.[7] While everything must be kept in perspective, youth and beauty provide a strong emotional foundation upon which we can recover. By aligning the external with the internal, Brazilians have achieved a unique, holistic approach to weather the storm.

Brazil —A Natural Environment for Youth and Beauty

Scientists estimate that approximately 20,000 years ago the earth was nearly covered in a sheet of ice. The Ice Age affected larger parts of North America and Eurasia, but scientists believe areas such as the Amazon forest escaped its wrath. As a result, the Amazon in particular and Brazil in general enjoy some of the most diverse plants on earth. In fact, over 250,000 botanical species are estimated to exist in the Amazon basin alone.[8] And with this diversity comes an array of natural chemicals and foods found nowhere else. Science is only beginning to unlock these mysteries, but even now, several substances important in slowing the aging process have been identified.

A few of these unusual foods common to Brazil are only now being realized as youth-promoting. Açaí berries found in the Amazon have been found to contain the highest amount of antioxidants of any natural fruit or vegetable. This little berry not only harbors important vitamins, minerals, and amino acids, but it also contains known phytochemicals that protect you from the aging process.[9] Maracujá, or passion fruit, likewise has an abundance of antioxidants and free-radical scavengers. These properties allow harmful inflammatory products to be neutralized in the body, preventing age-related damage from occurring.[10] Many substances such as Brazil nut oils and cupuaçu contain phytosterols and hydrating chemicals ideal for promoting smooth, healthy skin while protecting cells from sun-related damage.[11] It's no wonder Brazilians naturally appear so youthful and beautiful.

In later chapters, each of these fruits and vegetables will be described in detail in order to provide a better understanding exactly how these substances promote beauty and youth. The current knowledge about the aging process will also be explained so the cause and effect between Brazilian diet and health can be better appreciated. Regardless, Brazil appears to have been the fortunate recipient of the by-products of prolonged evolution. The ability of such a diverse number of plants and chemicals to evolve over time offers an advantage over traditional scientific efforts. Not only are such advantages less costly, but most of the time they are also more healthy.

Remember envisioning the sun-soaked sands of Rio and enjoying the ocean breeze? Perhaps a hike in a tropical rain forest would be just as appealing. Unlike many other places in the world, Brazil offers an array of environments all of which promote health and beauty. The fresh salt air off the ocean invigorates without the pollutants common to urban sprawls. The dense, oxygenated air of the rain forest energizes without the threat of carbon monoxide. While Brazil certainly has its share of urban centers, the opportunities to escape these concrete jungles and enjoy natural, toxin-free settings are abundant. Brazilians see this as a necessity and one reason they flock to the beaches when possible. Being able to avoid toxic substances is likely an important reason why Brazilians enjoy seemingly endless youth and beauty. Not only is Brazil aesthetically astounding, but it also does the body as much good as it does the soul.

With such a beautiful outdoors environment, it should come as no surprise Brazilians enjoy being physically active. While many of us require scientific study to prove the benefits of exercise, Brazilians have long realized the relationship between fitness, beauty, and health. As part of a culture proud of the human form, Brazilians invest significant time in sculpting their bodies and beautifying their physiques. Clothing is often scant as a result of the intense heat of the climate, and looking one's best on the beach always has advantages.[12] But additionally, Brazilians prefer action to inaction. Brazil has now won the World Cup in soccer five times, and the country now boasts 18,000 fitness clubs, second only to the United States in number.[13] And beach activities such as volleyball, surfing, and calisthenics have been commonplace for decades. In fact, beach volleyball was initially developed in Brazil. In essence, Brazil has been ahead of the curve for some time when relating exercise to beauty.

In nature, a delicate balance allows species to thrive. When it comes to our own health, the same applies. Brazilians have found this equilibrium by balancing work with play, activity with relaxation, and external beauty with inner brilliance. Whether by chance, by heritage, or by the influence of their surroundings, Brazilians have acquired many of the secrets relevant to beauty, youth, and health. Fortunately, we too can enjoy these revelations by investigating their behaviors and preferences and relating them to what we have learned through research and science. In doing so, we can achieve the same essence of beauty and youthfulness people from Brazil have enjoyed for centuries.

All Eyes on Brazil

Consider the following facts concerning Brazil in its international position today. Currently it ranks third among health and beauty markets in the world, behind the United States and Japan. In fact, Brazil is expected to surpass Japan in the next few years.[14] In the next four years, about a third of the increase in beauty product sales is expected to result from Brazilian growth.[15] And among the world's top ten fashion supermodels, three are natives of Brazil: Gisele Bundchen, Adriana Lima, and Alessandra Ambrosio.[16] It's no longer just the samba and bossa nova attracting the world's eye. Brazilians have built upon their natural beauty and youthful nature to evolve into something even more magnificent.

Here's the good news: Brazilian secrets for youth and beauty are available to all of us! While you may not be able to enjoy the tropical climate and everyday indulgences of Latin culture, Brazilian health practices can be cultivated no matter where you live. The benefits of an active lifestyle can be imitated even if the weather outside is less than desirable. Antiaging effects resulting from openness and creativity can be adopted in your own approach to life. And secrets for youthful skin previously hidden within the Amazon can be enjoyed in the most remote areas today throughout the world. By understanding these Brazilian mysteries of long-lasting beauty, you too have the opportunity to be healthier, happier, and more youthful.

CHAPTER 2

Natural Botanicals and Science: The Modern-Day Fountains of Youth

Seeking the fountain of youth and beauty is far from modern. Ancient Chinese sages proposed perpetual youth could be found in medicinal remedies.[17] Herodotus postulated such waters existed in Ethiopia, while Alexander the Great is believed to have searched for a magical spring in India just years before his death.[18] And Spanish explorer Ponce de Leon discovered and labeled a natural spring in St. Augustine, Florida, as the mystical legend.[19] Unfortunately, none of these historical proclamations has turned out to be necessarily true, yet we continue to believe a way to achieve eternal youth and beauty indeed exists. The only difference today is that science holds some of the answers, and these answers are showing great promise.

It's no wonder we seek ways to prolong our youth and enhance our beauty. Youthfulness is associated with vigor, energy, vitality, and sexuality. Beauty strengthens our self-esteem, our confidence, our opportunities in the world, and our overall outlook on life. In a recent survey, 14 percent of women over the age of 50 years felt their top priority in choosing cosmetics was to look pretty. Seventeen percent stated their top priority was to look younger.[20] Striving to protect our youthfulness and achieve beauty is as natural as being human. However, we no longer have to rely on fantasies and folklore to guide us in the right direction. The modern-day pursuit of youth and beauty is much more grounded in fact, not fiction.

The Science of Youth—Age Accelerators

While Brazilians may not have had all the facts science has to offer today, their lifestyles, behaviors, and environment provide them with the means to deal with age accelerators. For decades now we have heard about how genetics predetermine many things about our lives. Genes are attributed not only to features such as height and weight but also to our predisposition to disease, longevity of life, and even personality type. While genetics do play a role, they are not as significant as you might think. In a study following more than 10,000 pairs of identical and fraternal twins for over a century, researchers were able to determine that genes accounted for only 3 percent of the effect on life span.[21] If genes aren't the answer, what is?

There is an ancient Brazilian proverb that simply states, "Between the beginning and the end there is always a middle." If genes are our beginning and senescence is the end, then certainly factors exist in the middle that accelerate aging. Perhaps the most notable of these factors discovered in recent decades are free radicals. A first glance this may bring to mind a liberal, leftist political group, but free radicals are unstable atoms and molecules having the potential to damage cell structures and cell processes. Some free radicals are formed by our bodies' own cells during regular metabolism, but others are the result of external influences. For example, ultraviolet rays from the sun can result in free radicals in skin cells, while tobacco, pollutants, and exposure to other types of radiation can affect numerous organ systems.[22]

Free radicals (also known as oxidative stress) are in part the reason why our skin begins to wrinkle prematurely or why we develop delayed healing and recovery as we age. Free radicals have also been implicated in Alzheimer's disease, cancer, heart disease, arthritis, and even diabetes.[23] While this is one mechanism by which toxins cause cellular aging to occur, toxins can also cause direct injury to cells. Consider the potential harm direct sunlight may cause to cell DNA. Likewise, chemical toxins in the foods we eat and the air we breathe can result in direct tissue injury. Unlike Brazil's clean ocean air and the oxygen-rich Amazon, other environments may expose us to harmful toxins that accelerate cellular aging.

Diet plays a significant role in health as well as youthfulness and can provide both beneficial and detrimental effects. When our diet provides a wide array of natural vitamins, minerals, and phytochemicals, we thrive. Our skin has a wonderful glow. We feel invigorated. Our bodies are able to fight infections more easily. And we look and feel more youthful and exude natural beauty. But our diet must be properly balanced. While reducing malnutrition worldwide has increased our life spans greatly over the last century, too much of anything can be detrimental. Rising obesity rates have demonstrated evidence that poor diets cause declines in health and longevity.[24] Not only the quantity but also the quality of our diets is important in this regard.

In addition to chemicals in our foods, scientists have identified other age-promoting molecules in our bodies. The molecules have been labeled as advanced glycation end products (or their very appropriate mnemonic, AGEs). AGEs have been found to directly damage the structure of proteins in our bodies as well as other structures. Additionally, AGEs cause inflammatory reactions within cells by attaching to cell receptors.[25] These molecules have been suspected of playing a role in many chronic diseases such as Alzheimer's, heart disease, and arthritis, and reducing them has been shown to enhance wound healing, insulin responses, and longevity.[26]

But what causes AGEs to develop? Most of the time, AGEs are formed within our bodies and are directly related to the amount of sugar in our bodies. As glucose levels rise, sugar molecules attach to proteins and cause them to connect to one another. During the first few days to even a couple of weeks, this process is reversible if glucose levels are reduced. But if glucose remains abundant, the linkages become irreversible, thus creating AGEs.[27] Imagine a bag of candy canes lying in the sun. If you find them after a few hours, you can probably still pull them apart pretty easily. But if they have been lying in the sun for weeks, good luck! Like sticky tangles of sugar candy, AGEs wreak havoc. They prevent affected proteins from doing their job, and as a result, cells prematurely age.

With so much refined sugar in our diets today, the risk of acquiring AGEs has increased. With an increase in obesity, the presence of insulin resistance is also more common. Insulin resistance means the cells in our bodies do not respond well to insulin, and as a result, glucose levels rise. This then leads to increased chance of AGEs.

These glycosylated molecules limit cellular life span. In a similar way, emotional and mental stress have also been linked to reduced longevity, with hostility, depression, and anxiety having the greatest effect.[28] But how does stress cause our hair to gray, our skin to wrinkle, and our bodies to age? Is it just coincidence that President Obama's hair grays before our eyes? The truth is that emotional stress causes physiological changes in our bodies in addition to emotional ones. And the result of these changes accelerates the aging process.[29]

As stress advances, so do the levels of hormones in our bodies. If the stress is short-lived, these hormones allow us to react quickly to the threat. But if the hormonal response is prolonged, these same hormones cause aging changes to occur. Rises in adrenaline, norepinephrine, and cortisol over time are related to increases in glucose levels (possibly leading to AGEs), blood pressure, bone loss, and infection risk.[30] This of course fails to address the loss of sleep often present, which is important for body restoration. Interestingly, stress as well as all the other age accelerators mentioned have antidotes. In fact, many of them you will clearly see as being part of the natural and traditional Brazilian lifestyle.

The Science of Youth—Youth Promoters

While science is still early in the process of identifying which substances may be related to the aging process, much information has already been gained. The good news is we are living much longer. A century ago, the average longevity was fewer than 50 years, but today this figure has increased by 50 percent, to 75 years.[31] The average onset of lung disease, heart disease, and arthritis occur nearly 25 years later in life than they did decades ago. And the average intelligence quotient has been steadily rising over time.[32] While prevention, better medical care, and earlier disease diagnosis play significant roles in these advances, so have many factors known to promote youth and health…and, secondarily, beauty.

Research involving proper nutrition has made some of the greatest advancements. The understanding of how vitamins and minerals are vital to cell function has grown considerable, as has our knowledge of phytochemicals, which are micronutrients derived from plants. All of these elements are involved in normal metabolism as well as in the prevention of cell damage and injury. In considering free radicals and oxidative stress mentioned previously, many of these nutrients help absorb and neutralize these dangerous molecules, thus protecting the body from harm. Such compounds are collectively known as antioxidants.[33] Vitamins A, E, and C are common antioxidants, as are many plant substances.[34] Many of the natural fruits and vegetables native to Brazil contain even rare antioxidants that prevent cellular aging. In later chapters, discussion about these foodstuffs and other antioxidants will be covered in detail.

The same aging processes that affect the rest of the body also affect our skin. These include poor nutrition, free radicals, oxidative stress, AGEs, and stress-related hormonal imbalances. But the effect on the skin is important in one significant way. Were you aware your skin is the largest organ system of your body? Being the largest, skin naturally is one of the most obvious, telltale signs of aging. Youth promoters for skin thus include various antioxidants in our diet, including vitamins, beta-carotene, and lycopene. Also, certain dietary fatty acids such as omega-3s help keep our skins' outer layer strong while preventing exposure to toxins and pollutants. Also, retinoids are chemicals that keep our skin smooth and facilitate healthy cell turnover.[35] Once again, many of these youth promoters naturally occur within fruits, vegetables, and diets of Brazilians. Through science, their secret behind youthful, beautiful skin is slowly being better understood.

Diet and the avoidance of toxins are certainly important, but intuitively we realize exercise facilitates youthfulness and beauty as well. We know friends who routinely exercise and appear vivacious and physically fit. Likewise, science has linked exercise to better heart health, lower blood pressure, and better muscle and bone health. Even mice programmed to age prematurely can reverse their imposed genetic predispositions by exercising according to scientific study.[36] But despite this, the reason why exercise helps promote youth and health remains unknown. For now, we will have to look toward Brazilian culture and lifestyle for the evidence regarding exercise until science can unravel the mysteries further.

In Brazil, one of the most notable aspects of its culture is the importance of family. Often sons and daughter live at home well into their twenties and thirties. Even after marriages, families typically live in very close proximity to one another. Brazilians are also very social, often meeting new acquaintances walking down the street, while at the market, or even while pumping petrol. In other words, Brazilians enjoy a great deal of social support and demonstrate a healthy dose of emotional expression, both of which have been shown to promote youthfulness and health.[37] Rather than internalizing and experiencing hormonal changes associated with aging, Brazilians externalize and work through their problems with the strength of friends and family. This is just another means by which Brazilians embrace youthfulness and beauty.

A Brazilian Recipe for Youth and Beauty

As we begin to explore different aspects of the nutrition, diet, lifestyle, and philosophies of Brazilians, the age accelerators and youth promoters discussed here will be reviewed in greater detail. This will serve two purposes. First, you will be able to appreciate the rationale behind the behaviors recommended for enhancing beauty and youth and how they link to overall health. And secondly, common patterns will emerge, allowing you to see how internal health relates to external beauty. Youth, beauty, and health are truly holistic in nature, and the Brazilian culture and environment show how such uniformity achieves natural beauty. In the sections to follow we will understand the science behind the culture and how you too can pursue youthful beauty by adopting similar practices.

SECTION II

We Are What We Eat—Brazilian Diet Secrets

CHAPTER 3

The Crippling Effect: Foods That Make You Age

One of my friends is a health enthusiast. Actually, you may legitimately call him a health nut. After realizing the many health and antiaging benefits associated with natural Brazilian foods, he decided to adopt a more Brazilian-style diet. But even with healthy foods, too much of any one item can be detrimental. My friend, as it turns out, loved the taste of Brazil nuts, which are an excellent source of the mineral selenium. Actually, a single serving can provide nearly 1,000 percent of the daily amount required. After a couple of weeks of indulging his taste buds, he suddenly began vomiting uncontrollably. Not until he discussed his new dietary habits with his own physician did he realize he was selenium toxic. With a little more dietary discipline, he was soon back to his healthy self.

Unfortunately, we cannot always rely on our taste buds to always tell us what is best for us. Likewise, our tastes cannot accurately distinguish between which foods are healthy and youth-preserving and which ones accelerate aging. Some foods most associated with rapid aging not only taste wonderful but also enhance cravings for more of the same types of foods. Through science, we are beginning to realize the crippling effects of many foods in our diets that perhaps Brazilians have intuitively known for centuries. From refined sugars to trans fats, we are just scratching the surface on how foodstuffs link to aging and cause beauty to prematurely decline. In this chapter, three main categories of harmful foods will be considered along with the process by which they accelerate aging.

Sweets Don't Necessarily Mean the Sweet Life

Sugars essentially come in two categories: natural and refined. Both sources provide rapid sources of glucose, which our bodies use for energy, but natural sugars are often packaged with fiber, vitamins, and other nutrients, making the glucose less available for rapid absorption. In contrast, refined or processed sugars lack these other healthy components and are essentially in the bloodstream minutes after eating. This rapid rise in blood glucose lies at the heart of a premature aging problem.

When glucose levels are high, insulin is released from the pancreas so cells may absorb the sugar and use it for energy. But our bodies were not designed to handle such sudden increases. As a result, the amount of insulin released often overshoots the mark, which in turn causes most of the glucose to be absorbed by our cells, causing blood glucose levels to fall rapidly. The end result is a rebound craving for even more sugar to compensate for the rapidly falling sugar level.[38] If we react to this craving by eating more sweets, the process repeats itself all over again. This is not the dolce vita we truly want.

Refined sugars ultimately lead to an overabundance of glucose in our bodies, and a major aging effect related to excess glucose is glycosylation. A high number of glucose molecules in the bloodstream over time cause increased glucose attachment to a variety of protein structures. These create the previously mentioned AGEs, which interfere with normal health functions. For example, glycosylation to collagen (an important protein in our skin, muscles, bones, and joints) causes reduced elasticity. This results in premature wrinkles, immobility, and sometimes pain. Glycosylation to blood cells and immune proteins causes reduced ability to fight infections and inflammation. This leads to tissue damage and disease in some instances. Glycosylation has been linked to numerous age-related disorders, including Alzheimer's, atherosclerosis, hearing loss, and cataracts.[39] Suddenly those sweets are sounding less appealing, huh?

AGEs are in essence molecules that cause damage to important cell structures through a chemical reaction called oxidation. Because of this damage, cells are no longer able to live as long, function as well, or even regenerate themselves as often. One of the more recent scientific discoveries has shown that AGEs shorten important structures called telomeres. Telomeres are what allow cells to divide, and the shorter they become over time, the fewer number of chances cells have to regenerate. Telomere damage by glycosylation is thus a significant means by which longevity is reduced and aging is accelerated.[40]

Chocolate, donuts, and candies appeal to our taste buds because they provide the glucose our bodies and cells need for energy. But the concentration of sugar in these foods is incredibly high, especially when compared to foods historically. Likewise, they lack other important components, such as fiber and nutrients, that limit the rise in blood sugar. With a quick stop at the convenience store, the amount of sugar we can consume in minutes far exceeds what our remote ancestors ate in an entire day. Refined sugars thus not only provide us with rapid sugar access but also an overabundance of glucose for our bodies' needs.

Bad Fats: The Expressway to Aging

While excessive sugars can lead to glycosylation and age-related effects, too much glucose in the body also leads to increased obesity through its conversion to fat. When cells do not need glucose for their energy needs, they convert the excess to fat in order to store energy for later. Our ancestors didn't have a grocery store on every corner, so storing energy was important. But today, such storage is not nearly as essential, especially in developed countries. This reason explains in part why obesity rates have increased worldwide. Though Brazil's obesity rate is a third of the U.S. rate, the convenience of high-caloric food has had some effect on this otherwise healthy country as well.[41]

While glucose is one way in which we increase our bodies' fat composition, the ingestion of fats from our diet is likewise significant. Fats come in two main varieties: saturated and unsaturated. Saturated fats have many hydrogen bonds and are solid at room temperature, while unsaturated fats do not have many hydrogen bonds and are oily at room temperature. Between these two, saturated fats are more "sticky" and have been linked to atherosclerosis, heart disease, and strokes as well as elevated cholesterol. Therefore, limiting the amount of saturated fats has been recommended to slow aging and preserve health.

While saturated fats should be minimized, another type of fat should be completely avoided. Trans fats are fats that began as unsaturated fats, but in an effort to enhance their durability, they were hydrogenated (a process by which hydrogen molecules are added). Trans fats rarely occur naturally and have no nutritional value whatsoever. For this reason, many states have legislated mandates requiring labels and even restaurants to provide information about trans fats in their foodstuffs.[42] Most commonly, trans fats are found in packaged baked goods, margarine, potato chips, mayonnaise, and French fries. However, any label containing hydrogenated or partially hydrogenated oils can be assumed to have trans fats present.

What links trans fats to aging? In essence, three important effects occur when trans fats are consumed relative to aging. First, all cells are composed of a lipid membrane, which by necessity contains fats. Cell membranes are critical for proper functioning because they allow only necessary materials inside cells and prevent toxins and harmful substances from gaining access. Trans fats, because of their altered structure compared to natural fats, cause cell membranes to be poorly formed, less functional, and more susceptible to injury.[43] Like a breach in a computer firewall, unwanted entry and access are allowed. The end result is that cells die prematurely, thus accelerating the aging process.

Secondly, trans fats enhance inflammation throughout the body by affecting certain immune proteins. Prostaglandin E2, which augments inflammation, is increased by trans fats, while prostaglandin E1 and E3, which reduce inflammation, are decreased. Like a prison guard who suddenly relaxes the rules, chaos takes over and order takes a back seat. The balance is thus shifted toward greater inflammation throughout the body, creating a higher number of free radicals, greater oxidative stress, and more-widespread tissue damage.[44]

Finally, the third effect of trans fats, and perhaps the best studied, involves their effect on cholesterol and plaque formation in the body. By influencing how the liver produces cholesterol, trans fats increase the amount of low-density lipoprotein, or LDL cholesterol, and reduces the amount of high-density lipoprotein, or HDL cholesterol. This pattern favors the development of plaque on artery walls, leading to reduced circulation, increases in blood pressure, greater risk of heart disease risk, and increased occurrence of stroke.[45] These are hardly conditions that favor increasing longevity much less health and beauty.

Without any nutritional benefits and an array of harmful effects on health, trans fats have been recognized as universally detrimental to health and youthfulness. Are increased shelf life and preservatives really worth it? Some unsaturated fats are necessary for optimal health. For example, essential fatty acids such as omega-3s help protect your skin from sun damage, reduce acne, and enhance smoothness.[46] But diets heavy in saturated fats, and in particular trans fats, can markedly reduce your ability to enjoy greater longevity and optimal bodily function.

Carbs: Purer Is Not Always Better

Before discussing the good and the bad of carbohydrates in our diets, one point must be made. Sugars form the building blocks of carbohydrates. Therefore, all digestible carbohydrates are eventually broken down into sugar molecules so our cells may use them for energy. And yes, if we eat enough carbs we run into the same problems with glycosylation, insulin resistance, and fat storage, as previously described with glucose itself. Monitoring the amount of carbohydrates is therefore important so we don't trigger pro-aging processes detrimental to our goals.

The other issue with carbohydrates involves their complexity. For decades now, diets have changed to incorporate increasing amounts of refined flour, which has been stripped of most of its natural nutrients. Flour has since been marketed as being enriched, but the degree of enrichment fails to come anywhere close to the nutritional value of natural whole grains. Complex carbohydrates in legumes, whole grains, and vegetables contain insoluble fiber, vitamins, minerals, and other micronutrients. These help to provide cells the ingredients they need to function optimally while allowing a more gradual absorption of glucose into the body. This gradual absorption deters the rapid rises and falls of glucose associated with many aging effects.

In contrast, refined flour lacks these nutritious and protective elements. As a result, glucose levels can rise quickly when eating these simple carbs, resulting in the same glucose roller-coaster ride complete with insulin overshoots and rebound cravings. Ultimately, excessive intake of carbohydrates, especially simple ones, ultimately leads to obesity, oxidative stress, and inflammation, and this in turn leads to premature aging. If youth and longevity are what we truly crave, choosing the right carbohydrates in a reasonable amount is essential.

The First Step: Eliminating Pro-Aging Foods

While science has learned a great deal about the negative effects of certain foods on health and aging, many gaps exist. For example, just a fraction of the actual nutrients in fruits and vegetables is currently known. Of the ones identified, we know only a fraction about how they benefit our health. As described in this chapter, certain foods and their components are clearly detrimental to longevity and beauty. Cells are unable to perform optimally, and as a result they die prematurely with less ability to regenerate over time. Though our knowledge may be limited in scope, eliminating the substances known to be aging accelerators is the first step toward the youthful, beautiful bodies we desire. The next is creating a diet rich in youth-promoting nutrients, a practice Brazil has enjoyed for centuries.

CHAPTER 4

The Brazilian Bounty: Natural Foods for Youthfulness

We are affected by our appearance every day. When we feel less than attractive, we hesitate and become cautious in our actions. One of the most impressive people I can remember was a young girl I met shortly after I arrived in the United States. She was bright, witty, and charming, and she excelled in her studies. However, getting to know her took a long time because she was rather shy. She was plagued by acne, which had left her face scarred, and she suffered from a lack of self-esteem as a result. Like the wonderfully fragrant elaeagnus shrub, which is often called Ugly Agnes because it's so unkempt, she felt the same dichotomy between her external and internal features. Over the course of time we went in different directions, but one day we ran into one another on the street. I was stunned. Not only had her acne completely resolved, but the previous scars were also undetectable. In addition, her skin glowed with radiance, and her personality boomed with striking confidence. Was this the same girl I'd known a couple of years previously?

Indeed it was. In seeing such an astounding transformation, I had to know her secret. But her secret was hardly revolutionary or even difficult. All she had done was commit to a natural diet consisting mainly of raw vegetables and fruits while keeping other foods in check. Within a matter of weeks her acne cleared. And in a matter of months her scars faded. Not only had her appearance dramatically changed on the outside, but her beauty on the inside was also able to come forth.

If any doubt exists that health, youth, and beauty are linked to diet, hearing some of the thousands of testimonials to the contrary should easily sway one's opinion. For me, seeing the dramatic change in my friend was enough.

Understanding that natural diets rich in fruits and vegetables have an array of both known and unknown nutrients for the human body, access to having fresh fruits and vegetables is of course important. But Brazilians have an even greater advantage than simply easy accessibility; they enjoy some of the most nutrient-rich foods on the planet simply because of their natural environment. Several foods with unique health benefits grow selectively within the Amazon and are readily included in the Brazilian diet. Science today is now beginning to discover some of the reasons these unique foods are beneficial, but the proof is in the pudding. Brazilian beauty is a reflection of how such foods can prolong youthfulness and create long-standing health.

The Brazilian Bounty

Having discussed the important accelerators of aging and their mechanisms of action, revealing the secrets of a Brazilian diet can be described within this context. Foods of the Brazilian culture offer key ingredients that counter the aging process. As a result, diets including these nutritious substances can offer younger-appearing skin, vibrant energy, enhanced mobility, and simply better overall health. A bounty is being set before you. Now all you must do is partake.

Cupuaçu: Who likes chocolate? In many ways this native fruit is very similar to the cocoa plant and has a fragrance and taste reminiscent of chocolate. In fact, one of Brazil's favorite delicacies is cupulate, which mimics a hot chocolate drink made from this fruit. As a large, melon-type fruit, the cupuaçu contains a hard coconut shell with white pulp and large seeds. Many have described the pulp as tasting like a combination of chocolate and pineapple.

Cupuaçu contains theacrine, which like chocolate provides a stimulating and energizing effect unrelated to its natural sugar content. However, from a health perspective, its more-remarkable youth-promoting benefits stem from a variety of phytochemicals and micronutrients. Among the most potent are flavonoids and quercetin, which exist in high concentrations.[47] Flavonoids have demonstrated powerful antioxidant activity that combats the oxidative stress of aging, while quercetin has been identified as an anti-inflammatory agent with cancer-protective effects.[48] Lastly, cupuaçu is highly hydrating, increasing the ability for cells to retain moisture by 240 percent![49] Similar to the effect of cocoa butter, this unique property keeps skin healthy and moist, enhancing an appearance of youth and beauty.

Jaca Fruit: This fruit is jacked with nutrients! Sometimes known as jack fruit, this watermelon-sized fruit is the largest cultivated melon in the world. Once having cracked through its hard skin, you will find that the fleshy fruit has a slightly sweet taste bursting with nutrients. In addition to natural sugars and dietary fiber, jaca fruit provides good antioxidant activity, having large amounts of vitamins C and A. Vitamin C also aids in iron absorption into the body and boosts the immune system, helping fight off infections and cancers. Minerals, including manganese, magnesium, copper, and potassium, are also in significant amounts. The best part is that jaca fruit is fat free and sodium free![50]

From the perspective of beauty and youth, jaca fruit reduces the AGEs formed by providing natural sugars with fiber instead of refined sugars. Likewise, the free radicals and oxidizing agents that damage cell structures are better neutralized by the fruit's natural antioxidants. As a result, cells function better and live longer. And without unwanted fats, jaca fruit offers a tasty part of your diet that doesn't add an abundance of calories.

Moriche Palm Fruit or Buriti: You may have never heard of this obscure, central Brazilian fruit, but the oil from it is well known in promoting youthful skin. Buriti oil contains a host of protective agents including oleic acid, tocopherol, and carotenoids, which enhance the skin's ability to remain vibrant, smooth, elastic, and soft. But moriche palm fruit itself benefits the body in others ways. Often served as a jam, jelly, juice, or ice cream flavoring, it provides an excellent source of vitamin C, which as in other Brazilian fruits enhances the immune system and increases cells' life span.[51] More will be said about moriche palm fruit's effect on skin cells in later chapters.

Chayote: This fruit packs a nutrient punch! Common to the Amazon region, chayote is a pear-shaped, fuzzy, green fruit belonging to the cucumber family. When cooked, it most resembles summer squash, while it retains more of a cucumber texture when cold. In Brazil, chayote is found most commonly in salads, salsa, and soups as its taste is pleasant but rather mild.[52] However, from a nutritional standpoint, chayote is anything but mild.

Like other Brazilian fruits, chayote contains a handsome portion of vitamin C. But unlike other fruits, it also has a strong protein component with multiple amino acids. Minerals also include manganese for energy as well as copper and magnesium used to augment many cellular reactions. Rounding out its nutrient powerhouse is also vitamin K, vitamin B6, and folate.[53] With a naturally low sugar and fat content, this fruit gives a great deal of bang for the buck.

Brazil Nuts: To be clear, these are not local Brazilians enjoying themselves during Carnival. Brazil nuts come from hard fruit that falls from trees more than 150 feet tall and that can live to be up to 700 years. The fruit often weighs as much as four pounds, and despite its long drop, rarely does its hard shell crack open. You certainly wouldn't want to be struck by a falling Brazil nut as you were strolling through the Amazon. Within the hard shell lies approximately 10 to 25 seeds that boast a sweet, woody flavor, and Brazilians often eat them raw, although they may also be salted and roasted. As is the case with most fruits and vegetables, the best youth-promoting effects are attained in its raw form.

Did you know Brazil nuts have the highest selenium content of any natural source? Selenium serves as an important cofactor to an enzyme, known as glutathione peroxidase, which is a powerful antioxidant. Therefore, selenium helps the body's natural age-fighting mechanisms work more effectively. Additionally, Brazil nuts are rich in monounsaturated fatty acids. Unlike saturated fats and trans fats, these unsaturated varieties cause LDL cholesterol to be reduced and HDL cholesterol to rise, favoring reduced atherosclerotic plaque formation. Finally, Brazil nuts have large amounts of vitamin E, B complex vitamins, and numerous minerals.[54] In total, these nutrients serve to further antioxidant effects and strengthen cell membranes, which have significant youthful effects on skin, vision, strength, and energy.

Maracujá: We all know Brazilians have passion. Maracujá are smaller fruit that come from Brazil's passion flower. Being extremely juicy and with an abundance of seeds, maracujá can be either yellow or purple in color and range in size, being as small as a lime or as large as a grapefruit.[55] In Brazil, they are often served as juice, but they can be served in desserts, as a mousse, and even as a flavorful caipirinha. The seeds are also often used to garnish cakes and pastries.

Unique to maracujá is its high content of beta-carotene and lycopene, both of which are powerful antioxidants. Additionally, lycopene is believed to provide protection from certain cancers such as lung, stomach, and prostate. Maracujá also has a huge amount of vitamin C estimated at more than a third of one's daily requirements nutritionally. Finally, maracujá offers a high amount of dietary fiber as well as a source for iron, niacin, and potassium.[56]

Açaí Berries: Want to lose weight while simultaneously enhancing youthful beauty? A great deal of press has been awarded these grape-sized fruit native to the Brazilian Amazon. In fact, 42 percent of some Brazilians' diets consist of these berries. The berry itself is composed of a large seed and a thin pulp rich in nutrients. In southern Brazil, açaí is often served with granola, while in the northern parts it may be blended with tapioca. Additionally, açaí is now commonly used as a flavoring in ice creams, juices, and liqueurs.

Açaí berries have the highest amount of antioxidants of any other fruit or vegetable. Antioxidants consist of vitamins A and C as well as a host of phytochemicals such as anthocyanins, proanthocyanins, and flavonoids. And despite its high carbohydrate content, the vast majority of carbs come from healthy dietary fibers, as açaí are naturally low in sugar.[57] This combination of nutrients is one reason why açaí berries have been labeled as a great part of a healthy diet that allows weight control, antiaging effects, and beauty enhancement.

Acerola: Looking for vitamin C? Compared to orange juice, these small cherries provide 32 times as much vitamin C! This, combined with a generous supply of vitamin A and phytochemicals such as carotenoids and bioflavonoids, awards these small cherries a powerful supply of antioxidant activity. In Brazil, acerola are often used as jams, jellies and even baby food. Likewise, acerola smoothies are a regular treat and are low in sugar. In addition to its pro-health and antiaging effects, acerola has also been shown to lower cholesterol levels, reduce gastric acidity, and help digestion.[58]

For most of you reading about Brazil's array of unique foods, most of those listed in this chapter are likely new to you. Not only has access to these nutritious fruits and vegetables been limited in the past, but awareness of their health benefits has also been unappreciated until recently. Fortunately, many if not all of these fruits are now available in many markets and offer everyone the chance to pursue youth and beauty in a more natural and healthy way. For those foods not readily available, others options such as frozen foods and nutritional supplements exist, as do other natural food sources with comparable health values.

CHAPTER 5

Bridging the Brazilian Gap: Nutritional Supplements

The alarm clock goes off, and the daily marathon begins. If you're lucky, you have enough time to properly care for your skin, hair, and nails before rushing to the kitchen to grab some breakfast. And if you're really having a good morning, that breakfast will consist of a nutritious meal of whole grains and fruits. By the time you have arrived at work or gotten the children off to school, the daily list of tasks is mounting. For the rest of the day and evening, optimal efficiency is required, as is discipline, to stay the healthy course. Only then can you ensure that your diet is nutritionally complete without overindulging, and you can successfully find the time to exercise and manage your stress properly.

Unfortunately, this ideal scenario is often not the case. In our globalized and technology-enhanced world, demands for our attention and time make adherence to a healthy lifestyle challenging. Temptations abound. Fast food, processed snacks, stress-motivated sweets, and exercise-bailout opportunities are everywhere. Unlike Brazilians, who have an abundance of fruits full of health-promoting nutrients as part of their regular diet, we must more earnestly strive to eat nutritious foods while avoiding detrimental ones. It's no wonder over a third of Americans take multivitamin and mineral supplements in order to stay young and healthy.[59]

In order to cover the distance between the diet we need for optimal health and the realities of life, nutritional supplements are not only helpful but also necessary. The intent of this chapter is not to cover all the vitamins, minerals, and micronutrients needed through supplementation. Instead, the nutrients previously identified among common Brazilian health foods will be discussed as well as the amount of supplementation needed. With this information, bridging the gap between our diets and Brazilian cuisine can be accomplished when time is in short supply.

Omega-3s—Youth's Essential Nutrients

Understanding omega-3s is a little like trying to learn chess for the first time. So many health effects have been attributed to these polyunsaturated fatty acids through so many different mechanisms, keeping everything straight is difficult. In essence, omega-3 fatty acids are essential to our bodies, but unfortunately our typical diet overloads us with omega-6 fatty acids. The optimal ratio of omega-6 to omega-3 fatty acids is around 1 to 4, but American diets commonly provide a ratio of 20 to 1 or more. Because omega-6 fatty acids are in meats and vegetable oils, we bombard ourselves with these routinely. In contrast, omega-3s are mainly in marine and plant oils, of which we have less opportunity to partake. Brazilians gain access to omega-3s through fish oils but also through grass-fed cattle. Grain-fed cattle in contrast have almost no omega-3s present.[60]

When balanced appropriately with omega-6s, omega-3s provide a host of youth-promoting effects. They are essential to the production of several human hormones and are thus involved in cell division, clotting, muscle growth, digestion, and immune function. As an anti-inflammatory agent, they have been found to reduce joint inflammation, lower LDL cholesterol and triglycerides, and protect the brain from aging. While omega-3s are readily found in salmon, herring, tuna, swordfish, and flaxseed oil, supplementation is often helpful to ensure adequate supply. Recommended dosing for omega-3 supplements are between 500 and 600 milligrams daily of mixed preparations. One should not exceed daily dosages above 1000 milligrams.[61]

Flavonoids—Natural Disease Inhibitors

Also known as bioflavonoids, these plant chemicals serve to inhibit disease-causing organisms affecting plants. While this property is somewhat lost in digestion for us, flavonoids have powerful antioxidant properties, allowing them to protect a variety of tissues from oxidation reactions and free radicals.[62] Likewise, some flavonoids such as quercetin have been suggested to have several benefits ranging from antiviral and antimicrobial effects to prevention of various cancers. Anthocyanins, another type of flavonoid, also provide neuroprotective effects to the brain and aid in conditions such as depression and anxiety.[63]

Brazilians receive flavonoids in two unique fruits, acerola and cupuaçu. Other diets provide similar flavonoids in onions, apples, grapes, and various berries. But eating adequate amounts of these can be difficult on a regular basis. Additionally, flavonoids come in many different types and may have different health benefits on a cellular level. As mentioned before, science still has much to learn, especially about the numerous phytochemicals that exist. Flavonoid supplements vary greatly, but average daily needs have been estimated to be between 25 and 500 milligrams daily. With this in mind, 500 milligrams daily should suffice, and any flavonoid supplement should not exceed 1000 milligrams daily.[64]

This dosing should provide the added antioxidant, antiaging, and anticancer effects necessary to promote a younger appearance and a more vibrant beauty.

Carotenoids—A Family of Antioxidants

If you desire beautiful skin and a youthful appearance, carotenoids are important. When you think of carotenoids, think vitamin A-like antiaging compounds. Vitamin A, as will be explained, is one of nature's powerful antioxidants, and the carotenoids are often synthesized into vitamin A once in the body. Carotenoids, like flavonoids, provide pigment to plants but are also prominent components of chlorophyll and chloroplasts. Once ingested, these can be combined with oxygen (xanthophylls) or without oxygen (carotenes), of which the latter has youth-promoting effects. Of the carotenes, two have major health benefits: beta-carotene and lycopene.[65] As previously noted, Brazilian foods containing these micronutrients include moriche palm fruit, maracujá, and acerola.

Beta-carotene is commonly converted to vitamin A in the body, and research has supported its antioxidant power in reducing heart-disease risk, preventing cancers, and enhancing immune system function. In addition, beta-carotene through vitamin A pathways protects skin from damage from ultraviolet sun rays and helps rid the skin of discolorations such as age spots.[66] Lycopene, on the other hand, is not converted to vitamin A, but it actually has greater antioxidant activity than this vitamin. It provides similar benefits as beta-carotene but has been particularly effective in preventing prostate cancer.[67]

Carotenes are most commonly present in leafy green vegetables and carrots in non-Brazilian diets, with lycopene being found in tomatoes and watermelon. Dosages for beta-carotene supplements should be around 25 milligrams daily, not to exceed 300 mg, while lycopene ranges from 35 milligrams up to 75 milligrams daily. In order to aid absorption, these supplements should be taken with vitamin E, which also provides additional antioxidant activity.[68]

Multivitamins—A Focus on Youth and Beauty

Volumes could be written about the health benefits of vitamin supplements. Let's face it—vitamins by definition are essential nutrients. If we do not regularly receive them through our diet, then supplements are extremely valuable. In the context of anti-aging, only a few vitamins will be mentioned. These are the ones not only prominent in foods native to Brazil but also ones that offset the oxidative stress of aging and facilitate optimal cell functioning and regeneration. While all vitamins may need supplementation, these are the ones identified as being most effective at promoting youth and beauty.

The first group of vitamins essential to youth and beauty are those with powerful antioxidant potential. Vitamins A, E, and C enable cell membranes, proteins, and other structures to have protection from the oxidative stress of AGEs and oxygen free radicals. In addition, these vitamins individually play an important role in many enzyme reactions. For example, vitamin E enhances the action of insulin, reducing insulin resistance while also increasing memory ability by improving neuron functions.[69] Vitamin C improves iron absorption from the digestive tract and reduces melanin production in the skin, reducing discolorations.[70] And vitamin A augments skin cells by moisturizing membranes, allowing greater longevity, enhanced smoothness, and less sensitivity to the sun.[71] Perhaps of all the vitamins, these three are the most significant in promoting long-lasting youth and beauty.

The second major group of vitamins related to youth and beauty involve biotin and the B complex vitamins. Unlike some vitamins that dissolve in fats and can be stored in the body, B complex vitamins dissolve in water only. Therefore, a regular intake of these vitamins is required in order to maintain healthy levels. As a group, B complex vitamins are involved in a number of important cellular functions. For example, riboflavin, thiamine, and niacin are critical for the production of cellular energy. Folate and vitamin B12 are important for cell division. And pyridoxine is imperative for the metabolism of amino acids and proteins.[72] Imagine how rapidly our bodies would age if cells were limited in energy, regeneration, and metabolism.

Ideally, obtaining these vitamins through the diet is preferable. Nature, through fruits and vegetables, often packages vitamins along with important minerals and other micronutrients so their absorption and effectiveness is optimal. But adjunctive supplements help ensure we always receive appropriate amounts of these vitamins to enjoy youth, vitality, and vigor. However, one word of caution is necessary. More does not always mean better. Balance supplementation with diet to acquire healthy dosages of vitamins without going overboard. Too much of anything can be detrimental.

Minerals—Antiaging Micronutrients

Only in recent times has the importance of minerals regarding health been appreciated. These trace elements help many bodily processes by facilitating enzymes and serving as reaction catalysts. Numerous minerals thus promote youthfulness and beauty.

However, only a few will be discussed here that are prevalent among Brazilian foods and have more-important functions in preserving cell longevity.

Though selenium is not required in massive amounts for our bodies to function well, selenium is critically important in promoting youthfulness. By combining with proteins to form selenoproteins, this trace mineral becomes a superantioxidant, reducing the development of heart disease and cancers while augmenting our thyroid and immune systems. High amounts of selenium intake have been found to specifically reduce lung, colon, prostate, and nonmelanoma skin cancers.[73] Presumably, all these benefits have to do with its antioxidant effects. Selenium is routinely found in cod, tuna, breads, and other meats in the United States, but supplements up to 400 mcg daily may provide added benefits in preserving youth.

Like selenium, manganese preserves youth and beauty through powerful antioxidant effects. Most importantly, manganese is a cofactor for superoxide dismutase, one of the body's most important oxygen free radical neutralizers. Therefore, manganese slows the aging process in nearly every organ system in the body. Additionally, manganese helps with magnesium absorption, cholesterol and fatty acid synthesis, and the production of various hormones. Finally, manganese is important for the health of nervous-system tissues, augmenting memory, alertness, and energy.[74] While manganese is present in abundant quantities in Brazil nuts and jaca fruit within Brazil, ample quantities can also be found in almonds, hazelnuts, whole grains, and vegetables. Combining dietary intake with supplements can help reduce aging and enhance health, but daily intakes should not exceed 11 milligrams daily.

The last mineral of importance to Brazilian youth and beauty is magnesium, of which 70 percent of Americans are deficient.

Magnesium is the fourth-most abundant mineral in the body and is critical to energy production, glucose regulation, and functions of the immune and nervous systems. Therefore, a deficiency of magnesium can lead to increased inflammation, reduced vitality, increased glycosylation (AGEs), and reduced cognitive abilities. While dark-green vegetables are usually loaded with magnesium, diminished quantities in the soil account for the prevalence of this mineral's deficiency today. Likewise, refined grains remove the magnesium often present in whole grain foods.[75] Because of magnesium's widespread importance to the antiaging processes, supplements between 400 and 600 milligrams daily should be taken to ensure adequate availability of this important nutrient.

Scratching the Surface on Nutritional Supplements

Many other vitamins, minerals, and phytochemicals are important as parts of basic cellular functions and play roles in promoting optimal health. Clearly, we have touched on only part of the broad spectrum of nutritional supplements needed. But the above micronutrients have particularly important roles in slowing the aging process and in preserving skin appearance, energy, memory, cognition, longevity, and health in general. Likewise, in reviewing foods unique to Brazil, these compounds are more readily available within their native environments. Knowing these specific micronutrients and how to supplement them is thus worthwhile in our pursuit of youthfulness and beauty as well as health.

CHAPTER 6

Brazilian Cleansing: Detoxification and Dietary Toxin Avoidance

Many have heard of the extravagant celebrations and parades of Carnival in Rio, but fewer have experienced Brazil's second-largest parade, Lavagem do Bonfim. Lavagem takes place quite a distance from Rio along the streets of Salvador, Bahia, Brazil's first capital. Every January for many centuries, thousands have watched as an incredible procession of musicians, costumed attendees, and dignified women of the church travel a ten-mile course to end at Bonfim Church. Participants wear white shirts, and women carry white vases of perfumed water and flowers as they march in rhythm with numerous processional bands. Ultimately they arrive at the steps of Bonfim Church, onto which the waters and flowers are poured as part of a religious cleansing.[76] In fact, the word lavagem means "cleaning with water" in Portuguese.

The celebration is a reflection of Brazil's history and dates back to 1754. The ritual developed as an honor to the blended religions of Catholicism, brought to Brazil by the Portuguese, and Candomble, brought over by African slaves. While the procession is uniquely Brazilian in nature, the process of cleansing is universal. In most religions, ceremonial spiritual cleansing is periodically practiced to purify one from the temptations and pressures of earthly life.[77] In a very similar way, the impurities we acquire in our diets and through normal metabolism must be periodically cleansed in order to embrace optimal health. Regular practice of lavagem of the body should play an important role in our health efforts.

With this in mind, this chapter addresses physical cleansing from two perspectives. The first involves avoiding dietary toxins known to advance aging and cause poor health. The second involves dietary practices adopted from Brazilian ways of life that assist with detoxification and cleansing. By adopting these practices, we can enjoy our own celebration—a celebration of youthfulness, beauty, and health.

Preserving Youth— Helping Your Body through Avoidance

When I was a boy, my uncle had a beautiful wooden canoe. Painted a brilliant red, the canoe gleamed in the sun and brought me wonderful enjoyment on the water. But over time the hot sun caused the paint to fade, and soon the seams between the wooden planks began to widen. Because there was no place to shelter the canoe, the weather took its toll on the small vessel rather quickly. In time, water would seep into the canoe, limiting my excursions.

Like the canoe, our bodies are vulnerable to many harsh items in the environment. The more we protect them, the greater longevity and quality of health they will enjoy. Having identified many of the dietary toxins in modern-day foods associated with aging, our focus should thus be to avoid the very foods associated with them.

Naturally our bodies have inherent ways to detoxify unwanted substances. The powerhouses of our bodies in this regard are the liver and kidneys. Both organs play major roles in metabolizing toxins, metabolism by-products, and drugs, and then excreting them through either urine or the gastrointestinal tract. Additionally, our lungs and skin play more-minor roles in detoxification as gaseous wastes can be exhaled and sweat can eliminate other agents. Despite these various methods of natural detoxification, each system has its limits. With so many dietary preservatives and chemicals today, these methods can be overwhelmed.[78] As a result, cells become exposed to toxins they normally would not have. For this reason, limiting bad substances in our diets can preserve health and longevity.

While pollutants and other foreign chemicals represent common toxins in the environment today, these will be addressed in later chapters. In this section, foods that can be deleterious to health and advance aging will be addressed. As such, three main categories of foods are most important to avoid. In each case, the food itself is not necessarily toxic, but the reactions the food evokes in the body accelerates aging, deteriorates cell function, and causes unwanted physical changes. These three food groups include refined flour products, omega-6 fatty acids, and various kinds of refined sugars.

Refined Flour: Over the last several centuries, refined flour products have come to dominate unrefined ones. The benefits of refined flour over whole grains stems from the ability of refined flour to be used in a variety of bread products. But in the process, nutrients are stripped away from the whole grain, and fiber is markedly diminished. Even if refined flour is enriched, the nutritional and fiber value is tremendously less. As discussed previously, we now realize that refined flour is rapidly converted to glucose while limiting the amount of youth-promoting nutrients we need. As a result, glycosylation, insulin resistance, and oxidation reactions (all of which damage cell machinery) occur more rapidly.[79] Ultimately this overloads the body with detrimental by-products that cannot be easily processed and eliminated.

In contrast to refined flour products, whole grains offer high amounts of fiber and nutrients. Fiber alone is not absorbed by the digestive tract but instead acts as an osmotic agent to facilitate digestive movement. In other words, it draws waste products forward to be eliminated. This process helps with bodily detox mechanisms, taking strain off the liver in particular. The vitamins, minerals, and natural plant nutrients present in whole grains also help neutralize free radicals and similarly reduce the demands on the detox machinery.[80] If we truly want to be our best and remain youthful in appearance, refined flour products should be avoided. Whole grains help us keep our bodies not only afloat but also looking brilliant in the process.

Omega-6 Fatty Acids: As previously noted, an ideal omega-6 to omega-3 fatty acid ratio should be 1 to 4, but unfortunately, diets in the United States are closer to 20 or even 30 to 1 on average. This ratio facilitates heart disease through negative changes in cholesterol patterns and hormone regulation. In order to better protect our bodies, we thus need to limit the amount of omega-6 fatty acids in our diets. Omega-6 fatty acids are predominantly in meats and vegetable oils that are common in most American diets.[81] While an increase in omega-3 fatty acids will be discussed later, limiting omega-6 fatty acids by reducing fat-heavy meats and replacing cooking oils and butter with flaxseed oil or canola oil also helps.

Refined Sugars: In contrast to natural sugars in fruits and other foods, refined sugars are processed, allowing rapid absorption. Sucrose (table sugar) is detrimental enough, but fructose and high-fructose corn syrup are even worse since these have essentially no nutritional value. Because natural sugars are combined typically with fiber, their absorption is slower, allowing a more controlled glucose and insulin response. But not so with refined sugars. Rapid rises in glucose from these products mean increased glycosylation and AGEs, an increasing trend toward insulin resistance, increased conversion of glucose to fat, and significant rises in oxidative stress on cells.[82] The line "sugar and spice and everything nice, that's what little girls are made of" wasn't referring to refined sugars. These are the things premature aging is made of.

Dietary Detox—The Brazilian Way

While avoiding detrimental foods is a great beginning, we can also promote youth and health by including foods that naturally detoxify our bodies in our routine. Antioxidants, high-fiber foods, nutrient-rich fruits and vegetables, and plenty of hydration provide the ultimate recipe for detoxifying our bodies. Some detox diets promote fasting, massive fiber quantities, and abundant hydration only. While these provide colon cleansing and detoxification, these regimens can be quite stressful. Instead, detox diets providing a reasonable amount of high fiber and water along with solid nutrient support are not only more healthy but also more tolerable. Implementing this on a regular basis is much more palatable.

With this in mind, an effective detox diet should include healthy foods while keeping total caloric amounts moderately low. Calories should be maintained between 1200 and 1600 daily depending upon gender, body mass index, and level of activity for purposes of detoxification. Likewise, because high amounts of fiber help draw toxins out of the body, hydration is required to keep up with increased elimination of wastes in both the digestive tract and urine. This avoids dehydration, which can be detrimental to cell function.

Finally, an abundance of micronutrients allows detox organ systems the ability to perform optimally and to regenerate new cells over time. With this overall philosophy of a detox recipe, incorporating the following Brazilian foods into your diet can help you gain a more youthful and beautiful appearance while reducing your weight and enjoying better health.

Açaí Berry Granola: Açaí berries are naturally high in fiber and provide natural sugars instead of refined sugars. Combining these with granola allows an excellent source of whole grains and fiber, which aid detoxification. In addition, a single cup provides 200 percent of the recommended daily vitamin C. Along with other phytochemicals, Açaí berries supply the body with powerful antioxidants. And the best part? A single cup of Açaí juice is only 125 calories.[83] Combining Açaí berries with granola is thus healthy, detoxifying, and part of a good weight-reduction diet.

Salad with Raw Chayote: While chayote can be cooked, raw chayote provides greater nutrition and preserves its high fiber content. Being in the cucumber family, it is ideal for including in salads and may also be used in salsas and soups. Chayote has almost no fat and provides 3.5 grams of fiber in an average-sized fruit. Additional nutrients include vitamins C, K, and B6, and manganese.[84] On the whole, raw chayote provides a pleasant, mild, fruity taste with ample antioxidants, fiber, and nutrition. Plus, at 39 calories per fruit, no one will be ruining a diet with this Brazilian delight.

Acerola with Mango Juice: Though not quite as calorie-restrictive as some other foods, one cup of this Brazilian juice is still only 85 calories. The amazing benefit, however, is the high amount of vitamin C it provides, which is 1200 percent of daily recommended amounts. While the antioxidant properties of vitamin C alone are powerful, acerola also provides vitamin A, carotenoids, and flavonoids.[85] As a juice or as a smoothie, this combination of fruits provides antiaging effects while helping maintain hydration during detoxification. And if fasting is considered as part of a detox regimen, supplementation with this juice can be nutritionally beneficial during this period of physical stress.

Brazilian Rice and Pinto Beans: A staple among many Brazilians, this traditional recipe provides high amounts of natural fiber with a single cup, providing more than 25 percent of daily fiber requirements. This traditional meal is ideal in assisting with digestive cleansing while also providing iron, calcium, and other micronutrients, especially if natural brown rice is used instead of traditional white rice. As a routine dietary component, naturally cooked brown rice and pinto beans in a combination of 65 percent rice to 35 percent beans are low in calories. Calories per serving range from 120 to 250 calories depending on seasonings, and the dish offers a great source of protein and dietary fiber.[86] Combined with traditional Brazilian spices, this recipe can help you achieve your goals for both weight loss and youthfulness while still being pleasing to the palate.

Quinoa Salad with Toasted Almonds: Quinoa is a seed endemic to Brazil used as a grain and prevalent throughout the country. One cup of quinoa yields 15 percent of the daily fiber recommended and over 8 grams of protein. In addition, it is a good source of iron.[87] When combined with almonds, zucchini, bell peppers, and other vegetables, it provides a nutritious, low-calorie meal that facilitates digestion and bodily cleansing. If cleansing is not the primary goal, substituting almonds with Brazil nuts is an excellent option, allowing selenium (and its antioxidant effects) to be readily acquired as well.

As with any detox diet, ample amounts of water are recommended. The above dietary recipes that include traditional Brazilian foods can be added to other cleansing diets as long as the detox method involved does not include heavy fasting and aggressive colonics. Detoxification diets promoting more-modest reductions in intake while replacing regular foods with higher-fiber content meals can certainly accommodate these recipes. While their cleansing process may not be as rapid, gradual detoxification is less stressful to the body. As will be discussed later, stress can accelerate aging and cause a decline in cell functioning. Instead of adopting such an aggressive approach for short-term results, embracing a dietary plan allowing long-term health and youth is often more practical and tolerable. Avoiding detrimental foods while choosing a diet that facilitates detoxification is a much better strategy to attain these goals.

SECTION III

We Are How We Live—The Brazilian Lifestyle

CHAPTER 7

The Energy of Brazil: A Passion for Exercise and Fitness

The lights dim, and the music beats to a deep, rhythmic chant stirring your soul. As you walk through the club, you cannot help but begin to move with the rhythm, and Brazilian men cannot help but stare. Feeling their passionate, machismo charm surrounding you, you slyly glance their way, admiring what you see. Beautifully bronzed skin, chiseled faces, and sculpted muscles derived from the demands of work and the pleasures of fitness allure you. Is it your heart beating now or still the music? Immersed within the energy of Brazil, you willingly fall captive to the sights and sound around you. Here, passion and physique become one. Here is where you long to be.

The Brazilian physique didn't happen by chance but as a result of a long-standing passion for exercise, fitness, and the body inherent to Brazilian culture. From sensual, artistic dances to numerous physical activities made possible by a favorable climate, Brazilian youth and beauty became an iconic virtue. Only now are scientists beginning to understand how these passions for exercise affect the aging process and preserve youthful appeal. In fact, exercise is likely the most powerful tool in preserving youthfulness. Come, step into the culture of Brazil. Let your heart and soul embrace its rhythm as it flows through your body. Drink in the exhilarating feeling of a body in great shape. Through the energy of exercise, we invite perpetual youth and beauty. It's all here for the taking.

Some Truths about Exercise and Aging

Step back a moment from your physical passions and consider what science has to say about exercise and fitness. For decades, researchers have believed aging was largely determined by our genetic makeup. In ways yet to be understood, genetic codes had preprogrammed cells to slowly decline over time. Indeed, mice have been genetically altered to age twice as fast as their unaltered counterparts in support of this philosophy. However, these same mice now provide us with evidence that the secrets to aging are not simply genetic in nature.

Dr. Mark Tarnopolsky of McMaster University took two sets of genetically aged mice and forced one set to exercise on a treadmill three times daily while the mice in the other set remained sedentary. Interestingly, the mice that exercised lived nearly twice as long as the sedentary mice. In fact, they lived nearly as long as mice that were not genetically predisposed to rapid aging. Not only did exercise completely reverse the genetic effects on aging, but it likewise protected mice from losing muscle mass, developing cataracts, showing signs of kidney decline, and losing sexual organ function.[88] Being physically active doesn't just keep your buttocks toned and your waist trim. Exercise keeps us young both inside and out.

Consider what we know about the effects of exercise on aging. As previously noted, a sign of cellular aging involves shortening of telomeres, the cell structures vital to cell renewal. As these structures shorten, cells become less able to regenerate themselves. Stress has been found to be a key factor in accelerating telomere shortening. But when comparing individuals who are under equal amounts of stress, those who exercise seemed to be protected from stress-related telomere effects.[89] In other words, exercise equips our cells with antiaging power! The more we exercise, the more we enable our cells to stay young and healthy. And with more-youthful cells, the better we'll look and the more admiring stares we'll attract.

In addition to cell renewal, we can also help our bodies by reducing insulin resistance. When cells don't respond to insulin well, glucose levels rise, causing glycosylation and increased fat storage. No one wants more fat storage! Fortunately, exercise has also been shown to improve cells' response to insulin. In a study examining 136 obese men and women, people were placed in four different groups. One group did aerobic exercise, one resistance training, one a combination of both programs, and the fourth performed no exercise at all. When the trials were completed, cell response to insulin was found to be much better in the aerobic and combined-exercise groups.[90] Knowing what we know about glucose and aging, exercise helps preserve youthfulness by making cells respond to insulin more effectively. That means less fat, less AGEs and a hotter, more-youthful figure!

While we all want to be physically attractive and desirable, a youthful mind is also attractive. Not only does exercise and fitness give us the younger physique we want, it also improves brain function. Several studies show exercise to be an important factor in promoting positive mood and learning through a process known as neurogenesis. Neurogenesis is simply the formation of new brain neurons that facilitates memory, enhances mood, and increases our abilities to learn. Running for depressed individuals has been shown to have the same positive response as antidepressants. Exercise causes increased neurogenesis in specific areas of the brain known to improve mood and memory.[91]

Physical activity alters brain chemistry and protein structure, favoring new brain cell growth.[92] We are still at the threshold of understanding how exercise translates into youthfulness and cellular health, but a clear relation between exercise and a youthful mind exists. Exercise helps us look young, feel young, and even think young.

The advantages that exercise (especially aerobic exercise) provides our hearts and circulation are well known. Improved heart rate, lower blood pressure, and healthy shifts in our cholesterol levels are consistent benefits for improved fitness. But did you realize improved circulation also helps your skin? Increased blood flow to skin cells provides oxygen and nutrients that improve cell repair, cell renewal, and cell detoxification.[93] That means smoother skin, fewer wrinkles, and a healthier glow. Plus, exercise is a great stress reliever. Less stress means fewer contractions of facial muscles, which can cause premature wrinkles.[94] The secret of Brazilians' skin beauty in part lies within their passion for being physically fit.

From the inside out, exercise provides youth-promoting effects, keeping us feeling good and looking our best. Hair becomes silkier, and skin becomes softer. The curves of our youth return. Our minds become more vibrant, complementing our increased level of energy. And our moods soar as we embrace the perpetual feeling of youth.

But quality of life is only part of the good news. Exercise imparts both quality as well as quantity of living! Compared to those who do not exercise, physically fit adults over a twenty year period have one-third the risk of dying.[95] If you're looking for the fountain of youth, there's little doubt exercise is one of life's best-kept secrets!

A Brazilian Perspective of Exercise

The Brazilian lifestyle favors youth and beauty. The desire for beautiful physiques, combined with the vibrant energy of their pursuits, provides a perfect recipe for being young, attractive, and energetic. No wonder Brazil's passion for exercise and physical activities runs high. More than 8,000 sports clubs currently exist in Brazil, supporting the country's love of physical beauty and health.[96] Brazilian climates invite numerous outdoor activities including volleyball, tennis, basketball, rowing, sailing, swimming, surfing, and even hang gliding. In fact, Brazil was where beach volleyball originated. And having won five World Cups in soccer and hosting the second-largest soccer stadium in the world, futebol continues to be Brazil's most passionate athletic pastime. You have to visit only one of Brazil's many beaches to appreciate the level of pride Brazilians take in their youthful appearance. Of course you'll appreciate that as well!

Since Brazil's humble beginnings, physical fitness and expression have always been a part of its citizens' culture. Early inhabitants adopted a martial-arts style consisting of precision kicks, spins, and elaborate acrobatics. Known as capoeira, this form of martial arts looked more like an exquisite dance and has been adopted by many international fitness gurus as part of their exercise regimens. Capoeira combines a strong aerobic workout with Brazilian chants, drums, and rhythms, and may be the way to achieve that hot Brazilian body you crave. A single workout can burn up to 850 calories.[97] Capoeira naturally combines fun, passion, and exercise in a way typical of the Brazilian philosophy.

Let's face it. Sometimes exercise can be a challenge for us. Treadmills can become boring and monotonous even with the television to help us through the workout. Resistance training can provide muscle definition and weight control, but this can also become loathsome. However, Brazilians have found a way around this drudgery. Their inherent passion for life naturally incorporates high-energy activities with fun and social environments. Capoeira, Brazilian dance, and other invigorating activities provide Brazilians with this ideal combination. In each instance, exercise becomes exciting and a rewarding experience instead of a daily commitment. As a result, they not only stay younger and look more beautiful, but they also enrich their lives in the process. Isn't it time you started living the same way?

Life without passion is said to be no life at all. Passion infuses everything we do with energy. When we are passionate for our lovers, we think of all the ways we can express our love. When we truly desire to look and feel younger, we pursue those things known to promote youthfulness, health, and beauty. Brazilians have done this for centuries by tapping into their inner passions. Whether it's soccer, dance, work, or sensual pleasures, their zest for living underlies all of their activities. This is their spice of life and their secret to youth and beauty. Though perhaps best demonstrated in Brazilians' dedication to physical fitness and beauty, everything they do is filled with enthusiasm. And it's the same reason we are so attracted to Brazilian youth and beauty.

CHAPTER 8

The Brazilian Work Ethic: Staying Mentally Active

Do you remember your first car? I certainly do. As a twenty-two-year-old living in Brazil during the 1980s, my most prized possession was a Chevy Monza 2.0. To anyone else, the car was hardly impressive, but to me, the car was everything. And better yet, it ran solely on ethanol! The type of ethanol used to fuel Brazilian cars is not the same alcohol used in a caipirinha or mojito, but nonetheless this biofuel reflects a great deal about the Brazilian people. Being derived from sugarcane, ethanol fuel has been labeled as the most successful alternative fuel source for automobiles. In fact, between 80 and 90 percent of all Brazilians today power their vehicles with pure ethanol.[98]

Brazil did not always embrace such a green alternative fuel resource. During the economic struggles of the 1980s and early 1990s, Brazil found itself having to import large amounts of crude oil to support its own people. In an effort to reduce imports while also stimulating economic growth at home, Brazil passed a law in 1993 requiring all newly manufactured cars to operate on a mixture of ethanol and gasoline. Almost overnight, flex-fuel engines emerged and became the most popular-selling automobiles on the market. Today, the large majority of Brazilians not only operates their cars on 100 percent ethanol but likewise prefer it to regular gasoline. These changes enhanced domestic production significantly and catapulted Brazil's agricultural and technology industries to the international forefront. With passion and enthusiasm, Brazilians always find a way!

Since Brazil's inception in 1500, an attitude of resiliency and perseverance has dominated the country. No matter what setback or obstacle occurs, innovation and a dedicated work ethic characterize the Brazilian mentality. Through positive thinking and optimism, Brazilians have not only survived a variety of struggles but have also consistently come out on top. In other words, their quality and longevity as a nation depend on their ability to keep an open and creative perspective about their future potential. Brazilians are best known for their ability to improvise when times get tough, which highlights their ability to be constantly alert and receptive to new ideas. These inherent traits have served Brazil well, and in a similar way, staying mentally active also aids our ability to stay young and healthy. Science is just beginning to unravel the relationship between the mind and youthfulness, and this may one day help explain how the Brazilian perspective fosters health, youth, and vigor.

Linking Mental Activity to Mental Youthfulness

I think of memory the same way I think of hearing. The first time I fail to hear something correctly, I become concerned my hearing is beginning to fade. Similarly, if I cannot recall the name of something, somewhere deep down I fear I may be losing a portion of my mental capacity. With so many people suffering from dementia in the world today, one cannot help but be concerned when these seemingly inconsequential mishaps occur. Fortunately, we do not have to sit idly by; there are things we can do to preserve our mental youthfulness.

In the chapter on exercise and aging, physical activity was

shown to enhance circulation to the brain, enlarge certain brain regions, and stimulate learning. But is the reverse true? In other words, does being more mentally active preserve youthfulness and health? While the exact mechanism by which mental stimulation affects aging remains to be fully defined, evidence does support a relationship between an active mind and youthfulness. Some interactions are more direct than others, but in total we can enjoy greater youthfulness by being more mentally engaged.

Neurons, or brain cells, behave like other cells within the body when it comes to aging. They are vulnerable to oxidative stress, free-radical injury, mitochondrial decline, and reduced cell regeneration as time moves forward. Therefore, systemic efforts to reduce oxidative stress, glycosylation, and telomere shortening also aid our mental abilities. However, mental activity has also been shown to increase specific chemicals in our brains that protect neurons from age-related decline. In a very organ-specific way, stimulating our minds can slow down the aging of our brains, preserving memory and learning abilities.

One important brain chemical is brain derived neurotrophic factor, or BDNF. Doctors at the University of California Irvine demonstrated how active learning and mental stimulation among older individuals increase this chemical, and it in turn increases the number of connections among neurons within the brain. The more neuronal connections present, the greater is our ability to retain memories and to understand complex issues. As an additional finding, the researchers noted the normal slowing of brain waves occurring with age is reversed in the presence of BDNF.[99] Based on these findings, actively using our minds indeed protects us from normal age-related brain changes.

When it comes to mental activity and aging, a prominent belief is that we must "use it or lose it." Increased brain activity is associated with increased blood flow to the brain and the release of chemicals prompting new neuron formation. For years, scientists did not think that brains of older individuals had the capacity to generate new brain cells and adapt, but increasing evidence says otherwise. The more we use our brains by learning new knowledge and engaging in new experiences, the more youthful our brains remain.[100] In contrast, the more we shy away from learning and new experiences, the more we invite the normal aging process.

In addition to the "use it or lose it" theory, another important theory involves the concept of cognitive reserve. Where using our brains correlates with keeping our mental processes in good working order, cognitive reserve correlates with our ability to save up mental abilities for a later time. The more we actively use our minds, the greater knowledge and neuronal connections we build. As a result, we enjoy a surplus of mental capacity, which naturally buffers us from normal aging processes.[101] If we want to stay healthy and young mentally, exercising our minds on a regular basis is thus imperative.

Linking Mental Activity to Longevity

If we regularly run three miles daily over a long period of time, naturally our bodies adapt and become able to perform this activity more easily. Similarly, the effects of mental activity on preserving mental youthfulness are easily understood if similar mechanisms are in place. But can mental activity preserve overall youthfulness and longevity? In other words, can being more mentally engaged somehow benefit our entire body and not just our minds? Some research seems to indicate this is indeed the case.

One way of measuring mental activity involves surveys that quantify levels of curiosity. This is a natural state of enhanced mental engagement. In a study examining more than 1,000 men around the age of 70 years over a 5-year period, higher measures of curiosity were found to be linked to greater longevity of life. In a similar investigation involving the same number of women averaging 68 years of age, identical findings were found. After controlling for other variables, curiosity seemed to be the key ingredient, allowing some individuals to live longer than the rest.[102] Though the exact mechanism by which this occurs is unknown, the association remains significant.

From a different perspective, the opposite seems to hold true as well. In individuals who have less-than-optimal mental functioning, longevity seems to be significantly reduced. Average life expectancy today for most men hovers around 77 years of age, while women on average live a little longer, to approximately 82 years of age. However, individuals with a variety of mental disorders ranging from depression to schizophrenia live significantly less. In a study involving medical record reviews of more than 30,000 mentally ill patients, life expectancy was around 15 years fewer compared to expected life span. While researchers thought this discrepancy might be due to suicide, in actuality a higher risk for heart disease, cancer, and stroke were found.[103] A second study reported similar reductions in life expectancy for mentally ill patients and also noted liver disease and infection as being more prevalent among the mentally impaired group.[104]

Theories accounting for this reduction in longevity for mentally handicapped individuals involve higher frequency of risky behaviors such as the use of tobacco, drugs, and alcohol. Likewise, a lack of social opportunity and access to effective health care are other considerations.[105] But such indirect effects of mental activity on longevity and aging may be only part of the picture. Increased intellectual stimulation among dementia patients has been linked to increased longevity unrelated to secondary, indirect factors.[106]

Additionally, positive mental activity has been shown to reduce a host of physical illnesses and diseases compared to negative mental activity.[107] Clearly these indirect effects between mental activity and health do not provide the entire explanation.

While science lacks a complete cause-and-effect answer between the mind and the aging process, stimulating mental activity in some way lengthens life span and reduces other health disorders. In addition to protecting the brain and neurons from normal aging, increased mental engagement also benefits us in other ways, extending youth and improving overall quality of life. In time, science will likely reveal these hidden relationships, but evidence both from research and from Brazilian culture supports the benefits between an active mind and perpetual youth.

Staying Mentally Active the Brazilian Way

Given the evidence discussed in this chapter, part of our strategy to preserve youthfulness and health should certainly involve active use of our minds. For Brazilians, benefits have evolved through a positive attitude, optimism, a strong work ethic, and the ability to be creative and innovative. As a skilled surgeon, I credit my ability to perform under pressure in challenging situations to my Brazilian heritage. In Brazil, improvisation and creativity are cornerstones of success and survival. Through this, we exhibit our thirst for life and our passion to excel. And this mental energy provides the recipe needed to keep us young mentally as well as physically.

Scientifically speaking, active learning, new experiences, and frequent social engagements have been identified as enhancing brain performance and physical longevity. Therefore, incorporating these mental and behavioral habits into our lives should be a focus if we too want to enjoy a sharp mind and a long life.

As part of a prescription for achieving youthfulness and health, seeking opportunities to engage our minds is important. Instead of shying away from new opportunities out of fear or feelings of discomfort, we should embrace the opportunity as a chance to learn. Rather than being satisfied with the same old routine, we should pursue the chance to educate ourselves about new subjects and fields of study. And instead of listing all the reasons why something is going to fail, we should force ourselves to think positively about the outcome and verbalize that result often.

If you're looking for the common thread among these activities, it lies within a passionate thirst for growth. Brazilians have an intense passion for a better life and to attain the basic necessities to drive them forward. Whether it's financial security, better health, or simply better living conditions, *necessity* is often at the heart of their passions and drives. Ultimately, this keeps them mentally vibrant and allows them to enjoy the youthful fruits of their efforts.

CHAPTER 9

Brazilian Balance: Making Time for Sleep and Relaxation

Lost in a world of pillows and blankets, you slowly open your eyes. No alarms. No invading streaks of sunlight. The morning is yours. You snuggle against your partner, warming yourself from the slight chill in the air outside the blankets. Then after a few moments you gradually stretch, squeezing the grogginess from your muscles. You feel fully rested. Your body has been restored, and your mind is fresh for the day. This is the way every day should begin: relaxed, peaceful, tranquil. Not only do you feel recharged, but you also see the world around you full of opportunity and wonder. It's no wonder they call it beauty sleep.

Unfortunately these mornings are rare for most of us. The alarm does demand our immediate attention. Schedules must be kept. And though we attempt to steal as much sleep as possible, we feel obligated to negotiate these hours against daily responsibilities. Many of us deprive our bodies of sleep by choice, while others suffer a lack of sleep from insomnia. In fact, as many as 30 percent of individuals have trouble falling or staying asleep! The good news is we can have many more mornings like the one described above. All it takes is a commitment to attaining better sleep and adopting a life balance between work and leisure typical of most Brazilians.

While sleep, youth, and beauty will be discussed from a scientific point of view, it is noteworthy that Brazilians historically have adopted a much healthier lifestyle, balancing their lives between work and leisure. Brazilians indeed enjoy a strong work ethic, but they also make time for socialization, rest, and holiday. This, combined with a positive, fun-loving attitude, keeps Brazilians youthful and energetic not only in spirit but also in physical appearance. Brazilians have learned that all work and no play not only makes you dull but also makes you a little older and a little less attractive as well.

The Brazilian Attitude toward Work-Life Balance

Brazilians are passionate about everything. When it comes to work, they dedicate themselves toward achieving success through a strong work ethic. When it comes to family, Brazilians are deeply committed to maintaining intimate connections with relatives throughout their lives. And when it comes to leisure and fun, no other culture has more elaborate festivals, parties, or gatherings than Brazil's. For centuries, Brazilians have successfully achieved a balance between work and leisure. By keeping each in a good proportion, they have come to enjoy peaceful relaxation, adequate sleep, and focused energy.

Interestingly, this work-life balance has been measured and quantified. The Organization for Economic Cooperation and Development (OECD) recently compiled a list of indices measuring work-life balance for several countries. In its rankings, Brazilians were found to be above average in health and life satisfaction as well as work-life balance. Compared to individuals in the United States, Brazilians spend 30 minutes more daily on leisure activities. This placed Brazil in the upper half of all countries measured, while the United States ranked in the bottom quarter.[108] In other words,

Brazilians have a Better Life Index ranking better than most nations and far better than Americans.[109]

Three adjectives best describe the Brazilian attitude: happy, positive, and friendly. As a people, they are hard-working and energetic, but they approach every task with a smile and a good attitude. Rarely will topics evoking negative thoughts or feelings be dwelled upon. Instead, optimism rules the day, with the glass always being half full rather than half empty. Perhaps this healthy perspective of life comes naturally through their heritage, or maybe they have simply adopted a philosophy that works for their culture. Either way, this positivity strengthens their ability to achieve an effective balance between work and leisure. Their optimism permits greater efficiency in their work while also allowing them to deal with stress and challenges more effectively.[110] Because they allow themselves the ability to recharge, the best side of them shines through! You can enjoy this same positive outlook as well. All you need to do is rebalance your life by making time for the rest and relaxation you need.

Health and Leisure

Having described the Brazilian attitude and work-life balance, we will now turn our attention to what science has revealed regarding personality styles and health. Decades ago, distinctions between personality types A and B were considered important. Personality type A was high-strung, active, stressed, and always on the go. Personality type B was more laid back, sedentary, easy-going, and relaxed. Type A was associated with increased rates of high blood pressure, heart disease, and stress-related illnesses. But since then, science has identified specific traits within this personality type that are more relevant.

The most significant personality traits associated with reduced health are hostility and repressed anger. Both of these are linked to increased risk of heart disease. Additionally, increased blood pressure and cholesterol levels are more common in individuals with these features. Multiple mechanisms may be involved in this association, including a greater tendency to smoke, to overindulge in food, and to neglect exercise. Likewise, cortisol may play a factor in these risks since this hormone increases over time in relation to chronic stress.[111]

While hostility and repressed anger have negative effects, other personality traits have beneficial effects on health. For example, extroverts and people who are naturally social and outgoing have been shown to have 50 percent greater longevity than those who are not. Enhanced coping skills, less stress, and a stronger immune system are theories as to how this may relate to a longer life span.[112] Optimism is another advantageous feature. Optimistic individuals have a 50 percent lower rate of death from heart attacks and have greater capacity to deal with stress.[113] Finally, those described as being more relaxed enjoy a higher measure of life quality, have more robust immune system function, and are naturally better stress managers.[114] From these findings, it appears as if science is describing the Brazilian life attitude perfectly!

Leisure may also have benefits on health in other ways. Often we think leisure might lead to weight gain because we are less active, but what if it led to weight loss? In a study analyzing international surveys from over seventeen countries, a positive correlation between some leisure activities and lower body weight was noted. Reading, cultural arts activities, and leisure use of the Internet were all related to lower body mass among survey participants. This did not apply to those who watched television, listened to music, or socialized, however. The researchers concluded these specific types of leisure activity may be associated with higher levels of intellect and socioeconomic status, allowing them to make better choices about diet, exercise, and other weight-related factors.[115] It is important to note, however, that leisure itself was not a direct cause of weight gain.

Whether leisure enhances health through stress relief or other mechanisms remains unresolved. Regardless, objective evidence shows a clear relationship between better health and a more balanced lifestyle. Balance comes through moderation and knowing where to establish boundaries. In doing so, we allow our bodies to function at their best and adapt to changes and challenges most effectively. It's no wonder this strategy allows us to have greater quality of life and greater longevity.

The Truth about Beauty Sleep

We have all claimed to need beauty sleep at some point. Often our insistence for rest is simply because we feel exhausted, but can sleep really enhance beauty? Does lack of sleep accelerate aging? Does adequate rest promote youth? The answer to all of these questions is an emphatic YES!

Despite the many sleep specialists and sleep centers throughout the world, sleep medicine remains a virgin field of study. Think about it: unlike other fields of medicine, patients are able to describe their symptoms and physicians are able to see physical changes. But in sleep, patients are unaware of their experiences, and doctors must rely on indirect tests such as brain waves to gather data. It's no wonder we know so little about the effects of sleep on our health.

Let's start with the obvious. Sleep does enhance natural beauty. Even nonbiased measures to test this hypothesis have supported this fact. Recently, 65 untrained observers were asked to rank a series of images of 23 individuals according to their attractiveness, level of fatigue, and overall appearance of health. The 23 people had photographs taken both after a period of prolonged sleep deprivation and after a good night's rest. Even with the images presented in random order, the photographs of individuals after sleep deprivation were ranked significantly less attractive, more fatigued, and less healthy in appearance.[116] Without a good night of sleep, we clearly do not look our best.

How does sleep equate to beauty and youthfulness? Perhaps one of the common denominators is growth hormone. Interestingly, growth hormone is released in deep sleep. Deep sleep occurs cyclically three or four times throughout the night and is predominantly experienced in the first half of the night. However, deep sleep occurs as we gradually transition from lighter sleep into deep sleep. If we suffer from sleep apnea, poor sleep environments, chronic stress, anxiety, and other sleep-interrupting conditions, deep sleep may be significantly reduced.[117] Even when we choose to sleep deprive ourselves in order to accomplish more during our days, deep sleep is diminished. And along with it goes growth hormone.

Growth hormone promotes beauty and youth in several ways. Growth hormone helps cells utilize carbohydrates and glucose and in turn reduces insulin resistance, glycosylation, and conversion of sugars to fats. Likewise, it facilitates tissue repair and cell regeneration, deterring the development of cancers and other illnesses. Growth hormone also promotes protein and enzyme synthesis, resulting in better cell function.[118] All of these mechanisms counter normal aging processes, allowing youthfulness to persist. And when cells and tissues are younger and healthier, beauty is sure to follow.

These effects of growth hormone influence all tissues of our body in a beneficial way. In regard to our skin, enhanced cell youth and function mean collagen and elastin fibers are more resilient, giving our skin fewer wrinkles, greater softness, and quicker repair of blemishes.[119] Studies have shown that individuals who are sleep deprived have cells with a 30 percent reduction in their ability to process glucose. In this way, sleep actually promotes weight loss because cells are better able to access energy sources effectively.[120] In addition to increasing our levels of growth hormone, sleep has been shown to also enhance overall hormonal balance. Sleep-deprived individuals tend to have higher levels of the stress hormone cortisol.[121] Chronically high cortisol levels are associated with fluid retention, higher blood pressure, and higher risks for heart disease.[122] And fluid retention is one reason we collect bags under our eyes when sleep is poor.

With better sleep, we enjoy better cell function and better chemical balance within our bodies. When this occurs, not only does our skin glow and our weight drop, but our mood and level of alertness also increase. We become better able to deal with stress and become more productive. Memory and learning capacity increase as a result. We feel more invigorated, and we look more youthful. Even an afternoon siesta has similar benefits, allowing our bodies and minds to quickly recharge themselves. While many demands in today's world require shortcuts, we should never sacrifice adequate sleep. Beauty sleep is indeed a requirement if youth, health, and beauty are our goals.

Make Time for Yourself

While some Brazilians have trended away from daily siestas, many regions still subscribe to this leisurely practice. Recent studies have shown that 72 percent of some populations in the country take regular afternoon naps.[123] Certainly, the custom is common to Latin America in general. These practices, combined with attention to leisure activities, work-life balance, and a positive attitude, are strong reasons why Brazilians enjoy a wonderful lifestyle. Science is now supporting these behaviors as beneficial as well. We should take heed and learn to enjoy life, seek adequate rest, and relax instead of fret. With each smile, dream, and pleasure we add days to our lives. What's so bad about that?

What would it take for you to reclaim balance within your life? Would you need to assign responsibilities to others? Perhaps you might need to adjust your lifestyle in terms of work. When considering these measures, ask yourself what is most important to you. If health, beauty, and youth are your priorities, rearranging your schedule to allow adequate leisure and sleep is a must. Waking every morning feeling refreshed with a positive outlook on life can be yours to enjoy. All it takes is adopting a Brazilian attitude for life and a step in that right direction!

CHAPTER 10

The Brazilian Body: One Size Does Not Fit All

It's a beautiful summer day, and you've decided to walk along the waterfront, browsing store windows and popping in and out of different shops. As you begin looking at the latest fashion, a couple on the sidewalk grabs your attention. They are embraced in an intimate pose, caressing and kissing one another. The young man has gently pulled the girl close to his body with one arm wrapped around the small of her back, while she has submitted herself to his passionate kiss.

If the scene were on television or a movie screen, you would likely be enamored with their expression of love. But being the middle of the day in public sight, a part of you perceives their public display of affection as socially inappropriate. Now imagine the woman is also wearing a bikini and the man is wearing a Speedo, and imagine both are overweight and in their fifties. How do you feel about the couple now?

While the above scene may seem unrealistic to you, such occurrences in Brazil are quite common. Unlike many countries, Brazil's ideal body image does not conform to any particular shape or size, nor does body image dictate how people behave. Certainly, the world has embraced the Brazilian booty as sexy and curvaceous, and Brazilians do care about how their bodies look. But they also carry a sense of confidence and self-esteem, allowing them to be proud of their own individual physical appearance and unique look. They do not shy away from physical expression simply because their bodies are not tall, thin, and proportioned according to specific worldly standards. Because of this, Brazilians are able to enjoy who they are without the influence of others' opinions and judgments.

On the surface, having a healthy body image may not seem critical to youth, beauty, and health. But body image is extremely important because it drives many behaviors ranging from what we eat, how we exercise, and how we interact with others. All of these influence our health through nutrition, physical activities, mental health, and self-esteem. The challenge comes from shaking off what we have been socialized to accept as an ideal body and accepting a greater variety of physical beauty. Like Brazilians, we can attain a healthy body image of ourselves by focusing not only our outer appearance but on our inner beauty as well. When we do this, we make healthy choices, further enhancing our youthfulness and our true beauty.

Brazilian Culture and Body Image

In the 2002 film Real Women Have Curves, an eighteen-year-old Latino girl named Ana is confronted with conflicting images of what an ideal body type should be. Ana, who is young, shapely, and more full in figure, is perfectly beautiful and healthy. But she is constantly faced with the tall, thin, white, ideal stereotype immersed within the California culture where she lives. Not only is the pressure to conform to this ideal felt from her peers and the media, but even Ana's mother urges her to lose weight in order to change her appearance. The amount of self-confidence and courage needed to overcome these social pressures is tremendous, as Ana demonstrates in the film.

In Brazil, the pressure to conform to such an ideal is fortunately lacking. Stereotypically, Brazilians are seen as being shapelier in body image, but in reality bodies come in all shapes and sizes within the country. And no one is afraid to flaunt his or her physique! Whether at the beach or walking down the street, Brazilian men and women characteristically wear little clothing. Part of this reflects the climate during certain times of the year, but more importantly, their behaviors reflect their values. Instead of being concerned about meeting some unrealistic body-image ideal, Brazilians value authenticity.[124] They believe they should be themselves and dress in a way that best expresses who they are. In other words, they value inner beauty as much as they do outer beauty.

None of this means Brazilians care nothing for their physical appearance. The Brazilian wax originated here for a reason. But the key difference is self-esteem and confidence. In other countries, people shy away from showing their skin, wearing tightly fitted dresses, or expressing themselves in dance for fear they will be judged. They lack self-confidence to be who they are supposed to be. Brazilians certainly do not have this fear! Being a confident people, Brazilians freely express themselves physically and otherwise. This wonderful cultural trait empowers them to be natural, carefree, and passionate in how they conduct themselves.[125] And it allows them to perceive a variety of body types as truly beautiful.

During the Middle Ages, women who were rather plump were considered most attractive, vivacious, and healthy. With plagues and illnesses a bigger concern for the masses, a fuller figure was associated with greater health and beauty. However, during the nineteenth century, thinness became a more accepted body image ideal. For example in the United States, slender body types became associated with greater independence, control, efficiency, and success, all of which are considered positive character traits. In contrast, being overweight has become associated with laziness, a lack of success, a lesser intellect, and an inability to be athletic.[126] It's no wonder people fear being judged poorly if they cannot match up to society's ideal body image.

Fortunately, such is not the case in Brazil. On any given day, one can walk Ipanema Beach and see an array of body shapes and sizes all wearing whatever makes them happy and comfortable. Because this is the cultural norm, Brazilians don't obsess whether or not their waists are perfect 26 inches. Instead, they focus on eating healthy, staying active, and fully expressing their zest for life. With these things in place, body image will naturally reflect exactly who they are: youthful, beautiful, and passionate.

Body Image and Health

What image comes to mind when you think of the perfect body? For a woman, you might envision a tall, slender frame with slight curves at the waist and more voluptuous curves above. For a man, you may see a tall, muscular frame with six-pack abs and a prominent, square chest. These are common depictions within many societies of the ideal male and female body images. But a problem occurs when our own bodies fail to meet this standard. Can you imagine if every single person had these body types? How boring would that be! It would be like having chocolate ice cream every meal of the day. No matter how much you like chocolate ice cream, eventually it becomes dull and unappealing.

Regardless, many individuals become obsessed with this body image and even develop distortions of their own bodies in the process. These obsessions and distortions are at the heart of many eating disorders, including anorexia, bulimia, binge-eating, and even obesity. Did you know that 35 percent of all adults in the United States are now obese?[127] Likewise, 24 million people in America suffer some type of eating disorder.[128] Because the definition of the ideal body type is so narrow, many individuals struggle in coping with the reality of their actual body appearance. In the process they develop distortions of themselves in relation to this image. Ultimately this causes problems in their health and well-being not only psychologically but also physically.

Getting all the vitamins, minerals, and micronutrients our bodies need to stay healthy and promote youth requires a commitment to eating properly and taking supplements when necessary. But for those with eating disorders, supplying the body with optimal nutrition is a serious problem. For anorexics and bulimics, malnutrition results from inadequate intake as well as from purging after meals. Eventually, a host of vitamin and nutritional deficiencies develop, causing various organs to fail. The mortality from anorexia alone is 12 times greater for teenage girls than all other causes of death! Sadly, the mortality rate for individuals with anorexia and bulimia is between 4 and 5 percent.[129]

In addition to proper nutrition, mental health is also important to maintaining overall health. Stress causes aging to occur more rapidly by altering hormonal balances in the body, which in turn accelerates cell decline and impairs cell function. Likewise, as shown in Brazilian culture, inner beauty derives from a healthy dose of self-esteem and confidence.[130] Unfortunately, half of all people with eating disorders suffer from depression, yet a small fraction of these seek help.[131] Combining nutritional issues with low self-esteem and depressed mood adds insult to injury. Not only do these problems affect food choices, they also affect the quality of sleep, the level of energy for exercise, and the ability to handle life's stresses. As a result, individuals with distorted body images are prone to age more rapidly, develop health disorders, and suppress their true overall beauty.

Adopting Brazilian Ideals

Variety is the spice of life! We were never meant to look all the same. Each of us is unique, special, and beautiful in his or her own way. Therefore, why on earth should we all try to conform to a specific body type or image? Brazilian culture teaches that beauty comes from being ourselves, and Brazilians practice this in how they live. Instead of seeing themselves as independent, they sense they belong to their culture and community. They are connected to their culture and interdependent with others, which encourages them to contribute, share, and express. And because everyone expresses so freely, the tendency to be self-conscious and to judge others evaporates! Beauty thus becomes how well one fully expresses whom they are both inside and out rather than how close they conform to a specific bodily shape and size.

We are all products of our environment to an extent. Many of us have been socialized into perceiving certain body images as beautiful and others as not. Overcoming this tendency can be difficult, but the first step is to make sure you are pursuing the right goals. Instead of pursuing a certain weight or a specific measurement, commit to eating healthy, exercising passionately, and expressing yourself more fully. Talk to people. Laugh. Make friends. Seek ways to empower yourself and gain greater confidence and self-esteem. Identify your own self-ideals and values and match them with congruent behaviors and activities within your immediate culture. By pursuing these things, health and youth are bound to follow, and more importantly so will your beauty.

CHAPTER 11

The Nature of Brazil: Avoiding Environmental Toxins

While I was traveling along the Xingu River, a woman from the Kalapalo tribe caught my attention during one of my trips to the southern Amazon of Brazil. As I approached the village from a distance, she appeared young in age. Only later did I learn she was much older, and at 40 years of age, her beauty was striking. Her skin was a magnificent bronze and as smooth as silk. Her coal-colored hair shimmered in the midday sun. On a diet of fish, fruits, and cassava, the people of the Kalapalo tribe have survived in the deep recesses of the rain forest for centuries without the advances of westernized medicine, food preservatives, or modern developments. This enchanted woman embodied all the beautiful and youthful benefits natural Brazilian living bestowed.

Unfortunately, these same tribes are the ones being harmed by modern progress. For example, the health effects of the toxic insecticide DDT continue even today. Though DDT was banned in Brazil in 1997, its use spanned more than four decades, contaminating Amazonian rivers and aquatic life. While the levels of DDT in fish are progressively declining, recent studies have shown the toxin persists in measureable levels in these women's breast milk.[132] For a Kalapalo women who averages five children during her lifetime, this means ongoing exposure to an environmental toxin fifteen years after its last use! Despite the natural, youth-promoting diet and environment of Brazil, even here the avoidance of outside toxins are required to preserve health and beauty.

The Amazon rain forest covers some 2 million square miles and provides 20 percent of the world's total oxygen. Likewise, it contains over a third of all living species on the planet. It is the richest source of nutrients and health resources in the world, but scientists have barely scratched the surface of its hidden secrets regarding health, beauty, and aging.[133] Unlocking the keys to youthfulness and beauty within the human body carries similar challenges. But while we anxiously await each new discovery, we must avoid exposing ourselves to toxins and pollutants that negatively affect us. Like our efforts to preserve the pristine beauty of the Amazon, we must safeguard our own bodies from external harm.

Brazil's Environmental Battle

Many analogies can be drawn between Brazil's magnificence of the Amazon River basin and the natural beauty and youthfulness of its people. Through nature, both have flourished. But with progress, both have faced and continue to face serious challenges. In regard to the rain forest, DDT has not been the only toxin threatening the landscape. Other pesticides produced by major corporations have insulted Brazil's natural resources. Court rulings recently demanded Shell Corporation pay families and workers a sum total of $5 million for mental and physical health problems related to pesticide and smoke contamination of Amazon land and groundwater.[134] And progressive deforestation has eliminated 20 percent of Brazil's rain forest in the name of agriculture and development.[135] With the world's resources limited, efforts to take shortcuts and exploit opportunities in the name of progress will continue to pose threats to nature's health and well-being.

Brazilians have likewise been forced to deal with a variety of more-common toxins in recent years. As Brazil has catapulted itself into international economic and social prestige, industrial progress has naturally followed. Cities such as Rio de Janeiro and São Paulo are increasingly challenged by air and water pollution. And as a developing nation, food preservatives are more common, so products can stay on the store shelves longer.[136] Just as the environment of the rain forest must be protected, our own health must be preserved by avoiding an increasing number of toxins and pollutants all around us.

Fortunately, Brazilian passion and strength have been the force behind finding solutions to these environmental problems. In 1992, the first Earth Summit conference hosting 190 countries seeking global environmental solutions was held in Rio de Janeiro. Brazil was also the site for the 2012 conference.[137] Likewise, Brazil leads the world in green energy, with 47 percent of the nation's energy being renewable through ethanol, biodiesel, and hydroelectric resources.[138] And Brazil's president recently vetoed legislative efforts that would advance deforestation of protected Amazon regions.[139] This same passion to preserve environmental health should provide inspiration for similar efforts in protecting our own health!

Health and youthfulness thrive when our bodies receive the necessary nutrients, sleep, and balance they need. But at the same time, avoiding substances hindering cell function must be a priority. Toxic agents can accelerate aging and cause illness, limiting both quality and quantity of life. And when cells cannot function well, we certainly don't look or feel our best. Arming ourselves with a knowledge of what toxins are around us is the first step. Avoiding them is the second. While we may not be able to live in an environment free from all pollution, we can limit how it affects our bodies by making wise decisions. Like the Brazilians, we must adapt out of necessity in order to enjoy the beauty, youth, and health we deserve!

Pollutants and Toxins and Their Aging Effects

Form a health perspective, three primary pollutants and toxins pose threats to our well-being and youthfulness. These include the air we breathe, the water we drink, and the foods we eat. Air pollutants involve tobacco smoke and dirty air particles as well as aerosolized debris and chemicals found in emissions and smog. Even mold spores and infectious particles can become aerosolized at times. Water, on the other hand, is exposed to different pollutants. These may include agricultural, industrial, or sewage-related toxins or various organic and inorganic chemicals contaminating our water. And food toxins can involve a number of approved and unapproved unnatural additions. For example, chemical preservatives, genetically modified produce, and foods containing growth hormones are just some of the examples of accepted toxins in the everyday groceries we buy![140]

Because these toxins are unnatural and foreign to our bodies, serious health issues can develop. Consider air pollutants. In a study of more than 400 women age 70 to 80 years, the number of pigmented skin spots was correlated to known air pollution counts where each lived most of her life. For every standard unit increase in air pollution, the number of skin spots increased approximately 20 percent![141]

In a similar study measuring air pollution in more than a thousand people over a 19-year period, increased air pollution was associated with increased heart attacks and strokes as well as lung disease. Likewise, individuals in high air pollution areas had mortality rates 35 percent higher than those who did not.[142]

How do pollutants cause us to age more rapidly? In some cases the effect is a direct toxic effect to our cells. Research indicates pollutants and toxins trigger an inflammatory reaction because they are considered foreign substances by the body. In some cases, certain cellular proteins react to this inflammation by triggering premature cell death.[143] Fewer cells mean a reduced ability to detoxify other harmful substances and maintain normal functions. Aging is therefore inevitably accelerated.

While inflammation may cause premature cell death in one instance, it also causes the formation of free radicals and oxidative stress. Pollutants have been linked to a variety of health disorders associated with rapid aging, including Alzheimer's disease and Parkinson's disease. This occurs through oxidative reactions that damage proteins, cell membranes, and cell DNA. Preservatives, pesticides, air pollutants, and even heavy-metals toxins such as lead and mercury have been associated with increased oxidative stress.[144] And with increased oxidation comes increased glycosylation and the formation of AGEs known to accelerate the aging process.

Many foodstuffs today also pose serious concerns regarding youthfulness and health. For example, livestock fed growth hormone products to augment their size carry the risk of passing amounts of this substance into our bodies when we ingest related foods. Not only can this lead to hormonal imbalance, but it can also specifically lead to obesity and acne.[145]

Food preservatives used to slow bacterial growth also cause problems. Intuitively, these same chemicals also affect our own cells, leading to reduced function.[146] And genetically modified fruits and vegetables may also have detrimental effects on cell function. In many countries, these foods are not even allowed because their risks remain poorly defined.[147]

Through multiple mechanisms, toxins and pollutants accelerate aging and threaten our health. Fortunately, we know a great deal about many of the toxins and pollutants around us. Making wise decisions about the foods we eat, the water we drink, and the lifestyle we lead helps us avoid these aging effects. While we may not be able to rid our environment of every toxin, we can adapt the way we live to promote youthfulness and health. With a Brazilian attitude of improvisation, we can find ways to avoid these substances out of the necessity to preserve our health, beauty, and longevity.

Avoiding Toxins and Promoting Health

Having provided an overview of the extensive exposure we encounter today concerning environmental toxins, developing strategies to avoid them is certainly worth the effort. Think of the woman of the Kalapalo tribe whose body has been essentially untouched by modern-day chemicals and toxins. We too can look as beautiful and as youthful if we simply take steps to protect our own health. Here are a list of effective ways we can preserve our youth, health, and beauty by avoid potential bodily toxins:

- Choose organic, natural foods and seasonings when possible
- Avoid all processed foods and those with preservatives
- Avoid artificial sweeteners and artificial food additives
- Do not use plastics to heat foods in microwaves or store for long periods of time
- Use high-quality water filters
- Change air filters within your home often
- Get fresh air through outdoor activity often and regularly

- Practice proper care of skin, hands, and hair using oils, lotions, and safe cleansing agents
- Hydrate yourself well
- Perform regular detoxification behaviors

By adhering to these steps, you can avoid many of the potentially harmful pollutants and toxins known to accelerate aging and threaten health. Improvise the way you live according to the world around you. Adapt what you eat, drink, and do to the present environment. Brazilians have been adjusting to a variety of challenges throughout the centuries with astounding success. Today they continue to tackle such challenges head-on with the same can-do attitude. You can do the same when it comes to your health. Choose to safeguard your health and beauty by living a life free of toxins!

SECTION IV

We Are How We Feel: The Brazilian Philosophy

CHAPTER 12

An Expressive People: Brazil's Secret to Emotional Health

Even before she entered the room, he knew she had arrived. The slight breeze escaping into the party through the open door carried a scent of jasmine, which he had longed to be near many times. Standing in the doorway, she cast her spell over him once again. Her emerald eyes glanced around the room but eventually landed on his. But despite her hypnotic power, he looked away, fearful he may never be worthy of her magnificent beauty. He had to act. Why keep his emotions locked inside? Full of passion, he summoned his courage and moved toward her, but halfway toward his destiny another man intervened. His competitor whisked her away to dance, to laugh, and to love. That other man would eventually be the one she would wed, and he, sole keeper of his own feelings, would live to regret his indecision for a lifetime. The love he lost was the love left unexpressed.

Such a scenario could occur anywhere in the world, but the likelihood of it happening in Brazil would be less likely than most places. Between the machismo of Brazilian men and an overtly expressive culture, keeping such powerful emotions inside would be uncommon. Reflecting on his missed opportunity, the man who failed to act locked away his feelings without expression. Perhaps his broken heart led to resentment, depression, or a life of pessimism. Or perhaps he chose to ignore or discount his feelings altogether. In either case, his inability to experience his emotions, express his feelings, and manage them in a healthy and open fashion placed him at risk.

As we will discuss, emotional expression is linked to not only better health and greater longevity but also to a more beautiful appearance. From the inside out, Brazilians manifest their outer beauty through the natural expression of how they feel within. This is the lesson of emotional expression that we too can learn in striving to be youthful, beautiful, and healthy.

A Culture of Expression

A questionnaire administered to more than 15,000 business managers from around the world was examined to assess the degree with which managers from different countries used emotional forms of communication. Part of these affective ways of expression and communication included nonverbal cues such as touch, body posture, eye movements, and other physical expressions. After the data was compiled, countries were ranked from highest to lowest in emotional expression. Brazil ranked within the top five countries in the world![148] Of course, to anyone ever visiting Brazil, this comes as no surprise.

In order to understand why Brazil is so emotionally expressive, understanding the culture is most important. Unlike many countries in the world today that are individualistic, Brazil is better described as collectivistic. Brazilians place value and importance on the collective whole of their community, and in particular value family greatly.[149] This is much different from societies that focus on the individual. Their obligations to family and friends are not as strong, and therefore emotional expression is not as critical. But as a group-oriented culture, Brazilians have important obligations toward family, friends, and community.

Emotions are thus the means by which these relationships are established and maintained.[150]

Growing up in Brazil, I can attest to the fact that family is the most important facet of Brazilian life. Having the support of our families can make all the difference in the world. When things are not going our way, the emotional support from a loved one can determine how well we respond and handle our problems. Did you know that Brazil has one of the lowest suicide rates of any country in the world? While Russia has over 30 suicides per year per 100,000 people and the United States has 11, Brazil has fewer than 5![151] This data would suggest emotional support as well as expression may benefit Brazilian health.

Culture naturally affects personality, and the personality characteristics among Brazilians can be stereotyped using a few common adjectives. These include friendly, happy, positive, and inviting. Imagine walking into your bank or standing in line at a grocery store. If you're in Brazil, the person standing next to you will spontaneously strike up a conversation and engage you in a lively discussion. And before you leave, whoever may be around at the time will likely join in! Because Brazilians value family and community, they utilize emotion to endear rather than isolate. Because of this, they naturally migrate to positive emotions and shy away from the negative. In essence, they avoid conflict and criticism because these weaken social bonds.[152] Brazilians therefore are naturally more friendly, inviting, and engaging than people from other areas of the world.

The culmination of these cultural and personality traits ultimately provides the Brazilian people with a strong dose of optimism. The perspective that they can do anything, overcome any challenge, and improvise when needed evolves from a continual focus on what is good. And their ability to experience and express themselves fully allows their behaviors and actions to be saturated in this spirit of positivity. Even when things are going poorly, Brazilians look on the bright side. Because of this tendency and the widespread support received from family, friends, and community, they often make the impossible possible. This applies not only to everyday life but also to health, beauty, and longevity.

The Effect of Emotional Expression on Health and Aging

So Brazilians are more friendly, more expressive, and more optimistic. What does that have to do with being healthier and more youthful? Actually, quite a lot. A great deal of research has been conducted regarding emotional expression and longevity, and based on this research, five key emotional and behavioral factors have been linked to aging. These include emotional stability, openness to new experiences, agreeableness, a tendency to be outgoing, and conscientiousness.[153] In predicting which of these may impart greater youthfulness, it seems openness, extroversion, and conscientiousness offer the most significant effects. In a study of 70 individuals over 100 years of age, these personality traits were more prevalent compared to individuals who had died at earlier ages.[154]

It's quite interesting that the same traits exhibited by Brazilians are the same as those found living beyond 100 years of age. What is also interesting is that longevity is associated with the number of positive emotions one has on a daily basis in relation to negative ones.[155] But what makes us think positively or negatively? In considering what stimulates positive emotions over negative ones, genetics and life experiences play a big role in the process. A tendency to react negatively can be influenced by culture, environment, and a host of other factors.[156] But at the same time, increasing our positive thoughts can be a learned practice that in turn affects health and longevity in beneficial ways.[157] In other words, we can adopt a Brazilian perspective of optimism through more-effective emotional expression and attention to how we are actually feeling on a moment-to-moment basis.

How emotional stability, expression, and optimism allow us to stay youthful and maintain a healthier quality of life is not definitively known. Some research suggests the answer lies within the scope of cell renewal and neuroplasticity. Neuroplasticity is the mechanism by which brain cells reorganize and rearrange in an effort to meet life's demands. For example, learning a new language stimulates brain cells to restructure themselves in order to facilitate the new subject matter. Positivity, which invites new experiences, openness, creativity, and innovation, may trigger this process, thereby promoting youthfulness. For many years, it was believed older adults had little neuroplasticity, but recent research has suggested otherwise.[158] Through emotional stimulation, cells renew more actively and develop new patterns, helping us to adapt and to stay young in spirit. This theory has likewise been supported by research showing that greater emotional complexity (which comes with greater emotional experience and expression) increases longevity as well.[159]

Whether the ability to express our feelings more effectively and adopt an attitude of outward optimism enhances cell function has yet to be determined. But connections between emotional avoidance and declining health are generally accepted within scientific circles. In cultures where emotional expression is suppressed, avoidance can cause a variety of health problems. This may involve mental health problems such as depression or anxiety, or it may cause physical symptoms to develop. Believe it or not, physical symptoms from emotional avoidance are common. For example, individuals may have aches and pains when emotionally distraught or may even develop skin rashes when emotionally upset.[160] Even conditions such as psoriasis and eczema worsen with enhanced emotional conflict.

In Brazil, a holistic perspective of mental, physical, and spiritual health is readily accepted and practiced as part of health care. During my medical training in Brazil, clinical psychiatry was part of my curriculum four of the total six years. Psychotherapy is readily performed within the country, being preferred to medication. In fact, psychotherapists are required to undergo periodic individual psychotherapy themselves as part of their training. In contrast to countries such as the United States, where antidepressants commonly top the list of medication best sellers, in Brazil a greater value is placed on the holistic approach by investing in psychological healing through therapy rather than chemical treatments. Being aware of how stress can result in physical symptoms, healing the mind is a more targeted solution, providing long-term benefits toward comprehensive health.

While stress is one mechanism by which this occurs (as will be discussed in the next chapter), our emotions influence how cells and tissues of our body function. When we are emotionally drained, we often feel discomforts more acutely, and when we are happy, we feel our energy levels soar! As evidenced by how emotions affect the quality of our skin, it is of little surprise poor emotional health can affect beauty as well. Learning emotional stability, outward expression, and a positive attitude is thus very important toward our goals of health, youth, and beauty. It is yet another Brazilian secret we can easily adopt in order to attain what we value most.

Taking Steps toward Emotional Health

Keeping the friendly, outgoing, and positive attitude of Brazilians in mind, we too can enjoy greater health, beauty, and youth through greater emotional expression. But expressing our feelings may not come naturally. In order to accurately express ourselves, we must first be able to understand what we are feeling. The initial step requires us to actually experience our emotions as they occur. In other words, we must feel what we are feeling. Only then can we begin to express ourselves correctly and completely.

By allowing ourselves to experience emotions consciously, we invite the opportunity to then express our feelings to others. While the expression of negative emotions is certainly important to emotional health, this must be balanced with a positive outlook. As we begin to express feelings of sadness, hurt, remorse, or even anger, taking an inventory of positive aspects of the situation can help our emotional health greatly. For one, others will naturally migrate to someone more optimistic, and this in turn provides greater chances for emotional support.

While Brazil offers a culture that naturally fosters strong emotional expression and health, we can also achieve emotional strength by appreciating personality traits common to Brazilians. Be friendly, be outgoing, be happy, and be positive. And even when things don't go your way, look on the bright side while accepting how you feel. In doing so, you will provide your body with the emotional and mental energy to stay healthy, youthful, and beautiful. Besides, doesn't that sound like the way life was meant to be enjoyed?

CHAPTER 13

Brazil's Formula for Stress: Family, Friends, and Forever Young

Julia laughed until her belly ached as she sat among her family. She hadn't seen her cousin Daniel in several weeks, and she didn't realize how much she had missed him until then. The fact Julia was laughing at all was remarkable. Despite being 20 years of age, she had lived a great deal of life. At the age of 10, she had left her family to live with an upper-class family where she provided domestic chores for a place of shelter. At the age of 17, pregnant and no longer attending school, she returned to her family for support. And after the birth of her daughter, Julia struggled with several health complications, preventing her from working.

Today, with the help of her family, her daughter is well, and Julia now works in a restaurant near their home. And while life continues to be a daily struggle, Julia doesn't feel stressed in the least. In fact, she feels quite blessed.

Brazilians are not without their share of stresses. Income inequality, poverty, lack of a welfare system, and limited job opportunities are just a few of the common stresses facing many individuals in Brazil. But the specific stress is not as important as how they react and deal with stress in general. This is particularly true when it comes to health and aging. Different societies and peoples handle life stresses quite differently. Brazilians, having been subject to numerous challenges for centuries, have adopted effective ways of dealing with stress inherent to their culture. As we learned from the last chapter, their ability to appreciate their feelings and share emotions with others is an important strategy toward health and youthfulness. In a similar way, their methods of dealing with stress offer similar advantages. From the foods they eat to the inherent social support received, Brazilians have developed effective coping skills and strategies.

Stress and Aging

Let's face it—stress is everywhere. Time is short. Demands are high. Worrying about something is always an option. In a recent survey by the American Psychiatric Association, 75 percent of Americans worried about money, 70 percent about their jobs, 53 percent about their health, and 33 percent about their safety.[161] More importantly, more than half of those sampled reported personal health problems arising from the stress they experienced.[162] It would seem as a result of these reports that stress is increasing. The more stress we experience, the more problems we have, and all the while stress continues to climb.

Stress comes in a lot of different flavors, and similarly the symptoms we experience from stress are varied. For some, anger, irritation, anxiety and/or sadness may result from excessive stress. For others, fatigue, insomnia, apathy and/or headaches may result. The most significant symptoms relevant to aging and youth involve depression and obesity. Stress has been linked to increases in both depression and obesity in many societies, and once present, both conditions cause increased amounts of stress due to secondary problems. For example, depression causes fatigue, apathy, and sleep difficulties, which further affect job performance and relationships. Obesity affects self-esteem and self-confidence, creating poor lifestyle choices.[163] As a result, a vicious cycle of stress, declining health, and accelerating age develops, culminating in even more stress!

Specific to obesity and depression, stress affects health and aging through changes in the body's hormonal systems. Chronic stress causes persistent elevations in the stress hormone cortisol. Cortisol, which is normally released for short-lived stresses, allows our bodies to prepare for immediate action. For example, cortisol heightens our blood pressure, increases our heart rate, and mobilizes glucose for energy by increasing insulin release in the event of an emergency. But when cortisol is elevated all the time, these same conditions lead to chronic physical problems. Hypertension, heart disease, insomnia, and obesity become more common in such chronic stress states. Even depression has been associated with altered cortisol levels in the body.[164]

The presence of depression as well as other mental health conditions is important when considering how stress affects our health, beauty, and youthfulness. Depression as well as anxiety is associated with sleep disturbances, which affect optimal cellular function. Stress and depression often lead to poor lifestyle behaviors affecting diet choices and whether we participate in physical activities. Individuals suffering chronic stress often report increased television watching, consumption of higher caloric foods, and tobacco use as stress levels increase.[165] Depression has also been linked to telomere shortening within cells, which accelerates cell death and limits cell regeneration.[166] Stress and depression thus combine in multiple ways to accelerate aging, hinder beauty, and promote additional health problems.

While depression has been identified as a cause of telomere shortening, stress by itself has also been associated with this phenomenon. In a study of 39 women ages 20 to 50 years caring for children with either autism or cerebral palsy, telomere length in their cells was significantly shorter than in women without such stress. In fact, levels of oxidative stress were higher, and the level of enzymes required to repair telomeres was lower among this same sample of women.[167] However, it was noteworthy that only women who perceived themselves as stressed actually demonstrated these features of accelerated aging. In other words, the presence of actual physical or emotional stress was not relevant. The feeling of being stressed was what caused a decline in youthfulness.[168] From this we can surmise that our reactions to stress may be the more important factor than stress in general when it involves youth and beauty.

Stress therefore has both direct and indirect effects on how rapidly our bodies age, how youthful they appear, and our overall health. Through hormonal effects, cortisol and insulin levels become altered, resulting in reduced cell and tissue function. Through oxidative stress, free-radical formation, and telomere shortening occur, causing reduced cell renewal. And secondary factors such as negative lifestyle choices can lead to poor diets, toxin exposure, and reduced exercise. Given these insights, finding a way to manage stress in a healthy way is important. Examining how Brazilians manage stress can be very helpful in this regard.

How Brazilians Cope with Stress

Despite what many might think, Brazilians have a long history of dealing with stress. Throughout the nation's history, challenges confronted the Brazilian people, requiring the development of effective methods of survival. With each conflict, the Brazilian people became progressively better in collaborating and developing solutions. To a great degree, this is what forged their culture of collectivism and community.[169] Even today, in an environment of modern industries, the latest technologies, advanced education, and increasing urbanization, widespread challenges exist, and they cause many to experience stress on a daily basis. But because Brazilians are accustomed to improvising and surviving, people continue to flourish while preserving their health and beauty.

The most important strength of Brazilians in coping with stress involves their commitment to family. Similar to the benefits provided through emotional expression, having the ongoing social support of family and relatives meets critical needs when stress appears. Even after children become adults, they continue to stay close both physically and psychologically to their families. Most Brazilians continue to be a source of emotional and financial support for their children well into adulthood.[170] In countries such as the United States, the stress of being a caregiver for a parent or spouse is profound, resulting in marked increases in chronic disease.[171] But in Brazil, even as individuals routinely step in to care for immediate and extended family members, perceived stress is minimal.

Remember Julia? Could you imagine being in her shoes at 20 years of age? But with the support of her family, she feels completely secure, stable, and safe. Often, feelings of stress develop when we no longer feel in control. This is particularly important for people living in individualistic societies. Because the individual is responsible for everything that happens, he or she must control everything in the environment. It's no wonder stress is a problem for so many! But for cultures like Brazil's, the emphasis is on the group, not the individual. The need to control everything is not the primary focus. Instead, responding to situations in a healthy manner takes precedent. Brazilians have learned over time that the support of families and friends provides the best response to stress because it reassures them everything will be alright.[172]

When people feel more safe and secure, they become more comfortable in their environments. This prompts exploration, interaction, and openness. When people have adequate social support, they develop greater social competence and a sense of well-being. Ultimately, these things create communities of trust, sharing, cooperation, and collaboration.[173] In contrast, people lacking safety and security often perceive stress. If they also lack social support, the burden of that stress soon begins to place pressure upon them. If poorly handled by the individual, secondary issues occur, which can include a host of physical and psychological problems as previously described. It's not hard to understand why Brazilians have one of the lowest rates of conflict-related stress in the world.[174]

Brazilians have a common saying: fique tranquilo, or "don't worry." Imagine you were trying to hail a taxi in Rio de Janeiro. Just as you ran up to the cab, it pulled away into traffic. In some cultures, it would be quite appropriate to curse, scream, or make an unfavorable gesture to the cabbie. But in Brazil, you're more likely to hear someone say, "Fique tranquilo." Another taxi will be along shortly. In the meantime relax, have a conversation with the person next to you, and enjoy the moment.[175]

Effectively coping with stress involves managing our response to a situation. If we wish to be healthier, age slower, and enjoy life, we need not worry about the things we can't control. Stress is simply a perception. By understanding this and by reaching out to those who support us, we allow ourselves to feel more safe and secure. And this allows us not only greater peace but also greater youth and longevity.

CHAPTER 14

Spirituality and Youth: The Soul of Brazil

The warm morning sun awoke a magnificent field of daisies just outside the busyness of the Brazilian city. Amidst the flowers, despite their enchantment, a single daisy complained it was not receiving the attention it deserved. An angel came, trying to reassure the tiny flower of its beauty, but the daisy would hear nothing of it. It wanted to shine on its own. Appealing to the daisy's desire, the angel moved the daisy to the bustling city in the middle of the square. But a few days later, the city's mayor ordered the flower to be removed. The daisy pleaded for him to change his mind, but ultimately the daisy was tossed aside to wither. A single daisy cannot make a beautiful garden.[176]

This brief story summarized from Brazilian author Paul Coelho's blog uniquely describes how Brazilians perceive spirituality within their culture. As a society that values community, openness and sharing serve as cornerstones not only to daily living but also to the development of one's spirituality. Unlike many cultures where the discussion of religion is avoided in public conversations, Brazilians invite spiritual dialogue and are accepting of many different views of religion. Free from judgment or the need to have their views preferred over others, Brazilians enjoy a natural curiosity regarding their spiritual growth. This curiosity thus encourages personal exploration, deeper spirituality, and an innate sense of well-being.

Though ignored by scientific study for years, spirituality over the last several decades has been associated with numerous health benefits. Many theories as to how spiritual growth manifests better mental and physical health exist, but the exact mechanisms remain undefined even today. Despite this lack of understanding, spirituality undoubtedly leads to better health, greater longevity, and enhanced inner beauty.[177] The more we expand our spirituality, the greater the benefits. And for cultures such as Brazil's that invite spiritual exploration and interaction among its peoples, these benefits are realized more commonly. Brazil, as we will see, provides a rich and fertile garden in which spirituality and health can blossom.

Linking Spirituality to Health and Longevity

In order to appreciate how spirituality benefits our health and youth, providing a definition is a good starting point. Many use the word spirituality synonymously with religion, but spirituality in actuality is more of a personal pursuit. From this perspective, spirituality involves an individual's experience and relationship with a fundamental, immaterial aspect of the universe, and this relationship provides the individual with a sense of meaning as it relates to life in general.[178] As a result, the person experiences an inner growth that changes not only how he or she behaves and interacts with others but also his or her physical and mental health.

Over the past several decades, many scientific studies have linked greater spirituality to better health. In a cumulative review of more than 100 studies, 83 percent demonstrated a positive association between spirituality and health, while only 17 percent showed neutral associations. None indicated a negative relationship, however.[179] Specifically, increased measures of spirituality have been associated with reduced hypertension, heart disease, cancer, stroke, and colitis.[180] And in addition to reducing illness and enhancing quality of life, those actively pursuing spiritual growth in later years have half the rate of mortality compared to those who do not![181]

But how does greater spirituality improve our health and allow us to live longer? In short, no one knows for sure, but several clues suggest spirituality influences our minds and bodies in several different ways. Let's consider the effects of spirituality from a psychological perspective first. In studies surveying people's quality of life, mental health has been found to exert a much greater effect on their assessments than physical health.[182] The effect spirituality has on mental functioning appears to be twofold. First, spirituality increases the amount of social support available to us. For example, spiritual groups, church attendance, and belonging to a particular religion all increase social support, and as we have learned from previous chapters, such support benefits mental health as well as longevity.

Secondly, spirituality also increases self-efficacy or our sense of control over our environment. By gaining a sense of purpose for our life, we have less worry and greater confidence.[183] In some studies, existential well-being (or knowing that our life has a deeper meaning) has a more powerful effect on health than social support or behavioral changes associated with spirituality.[184] These effects result in reduced risk of depression, anxiety, and other stress-related conditions. Greater self-efficacy gained from spiritual growth likely promotes health and youthfulness in part by deterring the negative and age-accelerating effects associated with these negative psychological conditions.

The reduction in stress, anxiety, and depression by enhanced spirituality may benefit health and aging through mechanisms already described in this book. Spirituality may deter aging by reducing oxidative stress and/or by delaying telomere shortening within cells. But spirituality seems to have some direct effects on health and youthfulness also. Specifically, beneficial changes to our nervous system promoting health and youthfulness have been found with higher levels of spirituality. For example, the lowered risk of hypertension and heart disease among individuals with higher spirituality measures appears to be due to better regulation of autonomic signals in the body. Autonomic signals come from our nervous system and control bodily functions such as blood pressure and heart rate.[185] In addition, studies have shown that meditation and spiritual practices offset the normal age-related thinning of the brain's surface. This appears to occur as a result of enhanced neuroplasticity, the increased growth of new brain cells.[186]

From a scientific perspective, we have much to learn about the interaction between spirituality and aging. However, all evidence points to a positive association between spirituality, health, and youthfulness. Some of these positive effects may result from indirect benefits by deterring negative health conditions, but some clearly provide direct effects, promoting better mental health, physical health, and youthfulness. From what we do know, we should encourage greater spirituality for the sake of overall health. Instead of shying away from such discussions in everyday life, we should invite open opportunities for everyone to embrace spiritual growth.

Brazil's Approach to Spirituality

Brazil's culture concerning spirituality and religion is unlike many other cultures in the world. In part, much of this can be attributed to its heritage. Though Brazil's official religion for its first three centuries was Catholicism, the nation has since evolved into a multiplicity of spiritual practices. From Protestant to Pentecostal to several Afro-Brazilian religions, religious diversity is readily apparent. Through large influxes of immigrants over the last two centuries, Judaism, Islam, and Buddhism are also well represented. And with religious diversity has come openness, spiritual exploration, and acceptance typical of other aspects of the Brazilian culture. Because of this, religion and spirituality are important aspects of everyday social life in Brazil.

Based on the last census report, approximately 65 percent of Brazilians are Catholic while 22 percent are Protestant. Protestant denominations are multiple, however, and include Methodist, Presbyterian, Baptist, Jehovah's Witness, and more. A common religion also involves the teachings of Allen Kardec. Known as Kardecism, this religion incorporates many Christian beliefs with aspects of reincarnation and communicating with the dead.[187] Kardecism as well as Afro-Brazilian religions such as Candomblé, Umbanda, and Quimbanda reflect important aspects of Brazilian culture. One aspect is the tendency for Brazilians to believe in magical aspects of religion and spirituality.[188] This openness to the supernatural makes them more accepting and tolerant of its spiritually diverse culture.

One of the most spectacular examples of Brazilian spiritual rituals involves the Festival of Iemanjá. As part of the Umbanda and Candomblé religions, Iemanjá represents a deity considered to be the mother of all deities and goddess of the ocean. She symbolizes unity, family, and children, which makes her particularly important to Brazilian culture. Every New Year's Eve at midnight, followers of the religion and commemorators alike flock to the beaches in Rio de Janeiro all dressed in white. Holes are dug in the sand and filled with flowers and lit candles. Then at midnight, small, wooden boats are launched into the ocean filled with perfumes, combs, soaps, and candles in hopes Iemanjá will grant her devotees' wishes for the upcoming year.[189] This truly magnificent tradition highlights Brazilian mysticism.

The Festival of Iemanjá also demonstrates a Brazilian practice of syncretism. Syncretism is the practice of blending religions together to achieve a more personalized spiritual practice. For example, many of the Afro-Brazilian religions blended aspects of Yoruba spiritual beliefs with those of Catholicism during Brazil's early heritage. To an extent, this occurs with the Festival of Iemanjá. Natives and African slaves adopted these blends as a means to tailor belief systems and personal spiritual growth to their new environment.[190] Unlike many countries where religious beliefs and structures are more formal, Brazilians practice more-personalized rituals.[191] The uniqueness and personalized nature of these beliefs fosters a greater sense of well-being and purpose for each individual.

The power of spirituality comes from its power of hope and protection a greater power offers. Brazilians believe strongly in such supernatural powers, and through dedicated beliefs and practices they realize the blessings and guidance this power provides in their lives. Interestingly, Brazilians have been able to assimilate many religions within their culture because all are based on a foundation of hope. The saints of Umbanda correspond to the saints of Catholicism. Therefore, one religion is not at the expense of another within the culture. Assimilation is preferred over competition. In this way, spiritual support is valued just as social support from fellow Brazilians is. Spirituality becomes another means by which community, collectivism, and health are attained.

Combined with its more personalized spiritual practices, Brazil culture also enjoys an openness of religions among its people. For example, Brazilians routinely incorporate spiritual traditions in the workplace and individualize them to their own unique beliefs.[192] In addition, interviews involving more than two dozen Brazilian therapists demonstrated the use of spirituality was practiced both for patient purposes and for coping strategies for therapists.[193] Religion and religious symbols are also accepted and even taught within Brazilian schools.[194] Such integration of spirituality within every fiber of Brazilian culture contrasts with how religion is treated in many other countries. But instead of polarizing individuals, this practice in Brazil promotes tolerance, openness, and spiritual exploration.

As time moves forward, the mechanisms by which spirituality influences health will slowly be revealed, but even now we know increased spirituality provides numerous benefits to our health. Therefore, adopting a mindset of spiritual growth is well aligned with our goals of becoming healthier and more youthful. Brazil has developed a culture that promotes spirituality and personal growth by accepting a wide diversity of religious beliefs and practices. Additionally, the presence of spiritual discussions and practices in all aspects of their society encourages this further. While we may not be able to influence the culture in which we live in such a large way, we can appreciate the openness and tolerance Brazilians enjoy. By adopting a Brazilian philosophy of spirituality and pursuing our own spiritual growth, we too can enjoy greater health and youth.

CHAPTER 15

Desire for Beauty: Is It All about Sex?

Passers-by paused for a moment as she stepped out of the limousine. Her cascading, dark hair feathered across her shoulders, outlining the strength of her face, and her pale-green eyes offered a depth only the courageous would explore. Her long, slender legs, which had momentarily escaped the confines of her evening gown, slowly slid back into place as she stood before the crowd. From head to toe she exuded beauty. Even adornments of diamonds were perfectly placed to ensure her magnificence was revered. As she proceeded to enter the event, she could feel the heat of his gaze as it traveled across the curves of her body. And though she absorbed his admiration like a sponge, she refrained from revealing the moment's pleasure. She had him exactly where she wanted him…and he knew it.

Is there any doubt sexuality and beauty are intimately connected? Certainly, beauty can be appreciated in a great many circumstances that have nothing to do with sex appeal. But what drives us to become beautiful? Why do we desire to be the ideal height and weight, to have the right curves in the right places, and to attract the admiration of others who see us? As is the case with many complex questions, a single answer does not exist, but indeed sexuality plays a significant role in our desire. Different cultures value beauty as well as sexuality in different ways and to different extents. What may be beautiful and sensual in one country may not be so in the next. But ultimately, everyone wishes to be attractive to others. This is an inherent part of human nature.

In this chapter we will explore the motivations for being beautiful and the relationship sexuality plays in this desire. Interestingly, the motivations for Brazilians to attain beauty differ to a degree from other cultures, although some common themes exist. By delving into Brazil's history and current culture, a better understanding of beauty and sexuality can be gained. At the same time, comparing motivations for beauty in Brazil to other countries can provide a more comprehensive understanding of how beauty and sexuality interact. And with this understanding, we can embrace why we naturally have a desire to be physically attractive.

Health, Beauty, and Sex

Beauty is in the eye of the beholder, it is often said. Certainly, this is true as different individuals find varying attributes pleasing to the eye. Among different cultures, different body shapes, styles, and characteristics are deemed more beautiful than others. For example, thinness has been a core attribute of beauty in many westernized cultures since the mid-twentieth century, but in others, a more voluptuous figure is attractive.[195] The definition of beautiful even changes over time within a culture. This explains why the Brazilian physique is becoming increasingly popular within the U.S. culture. With this in mind, defining beauty is impossible unless we take into account the surrounding culture.

Beauty is of course made up of several elements. For example, facial attractiveness is a core feature of beauty in most cultures. At the same time, social charm, energy, personality, and confidence also play a role. And increasingly, fashionable style can go a long way in determining beauty. But perhaps more than anything else, sexuality represents a major component. The shape of our figures, the definition of our physical features, how we move, how we speak, and the degree of flirtatious playfulness all influence sexuality in addition to basic appearance.[196] Because of this, sexuality and beauty are interconnected. Beauty enhances our ability to exhibit our sexuality, while sexuality showcases our physical attractiveness in different ways.

Appreciating the interplay between beauty and sexual appeal, one important question remains. Do we desire beauty in order to be sexier? If so, then what is our motivation to be sexier? As usual, these answers are far from straightforward, and different opinions abound regarding the answers. For example, Naomi Wolf, the best-selling author of *The Beauty Myth*, would argue that the definition of beauty has been created and enforced by a male-dominant society as a means to repress women's equality. In other words, by requiring women (more than men) to attain some standard of beauty based on social expectations, women are kept at a disadvantage. The standard of beauty is then applied to a variety of circumstances such as employment and politics, limiting the ability for women to attain gender equality.[197]

Many disagree with Wolf's assessment of beauty. Scientific research examining a variety of cultures has found that attractiveness is most often attributed to the female gender even in societies where gender equality is well represented. The prevalence of this suggests the assignment of beauty to women more than men is evolutionary in origin rather than being based on social or cultural pressures.[198] In weighing these different opinions in the balance, perhaps the best way to perceive beauty is through a more practical lens. By incorporating the sexual aspect of beauty in the equation, beauty can be viewed as erotic capital or assets.[199] And like any other type of valuable commodity, erotic capital can be used as a means of influence and power.

If we consider sexuality and beauty as erotic capital, we can begin to appreciate why beauty is such a desirable feature. Gender differences have been consistently found between men and women in their desire for sex. Men desire sex to a much greater extent than women as a general rule. Especially after child-bearing age, men's sexual desire typically remains relatively constant, while women's often declines.[200] Studies have shown that men are twice as likely as women to have affairs. In Spain, 25 percent of all men have been involved with sex-related services at some time, while only 1 percent of women have.[201] While inherent social factors also play a part in this statistic, gender discrepancy in the value of sex certainly exists. This imbalance establishes the basis by which erotic capital can be a source of influence.

In a large survey of more than 37 countries on more than 5 continents, a consistent trend found women sought male partners who were economically strong, while men primarily sought female partners who were physically attractive.[202] Women also tend to be attracted to the romantic and emotional side, while men tend to be more hedonistic.[203] For women, beauty is an attribute that has value within societies. With greater beauty and sexuality, the opportunity for upward social mobility is more likely. This not only influences relationships over time, but beauty also influences other economic opportunities. In multiple studies, plain-looking individuals earn less than average-looking people, and average-looking people earn less than attractive people.[204] These findings persist even after other variables such as age, education, experience, and personality are considered. It pays to be beautiful!

So how does this all tie together? Whether a result of evolution or social change, beauty is consistently assigned to women as an attribute more than it is to men. And beauty, while composed of many features, cannot be considered in total without including sexuality and sex appeal. Because sex and physical attraction are valued differently by different individuals, beauty thus becomes a commodity used as a means to attain other valuable items. Ultimately, this means that enhanced beauty provides opportunities for better relationships, better careers, and better lifestyles. And with better social status typically comes opportunities for better health. Traditionally (and commonly in westernized cultures), the desire for beauty is intricately connected to sexuality and an enhanced lifestyle. Brazilians are no different in this regard; however, the perspective of beauty in relation to overall health is quite different. It is this additional perspective that makes Brazilians' approach to beauty unique.

Beauty from a Brazilian Point of View

Like other cultures, the Brazilian culture rewards beauty through greater social opportunities. In fact, Brazilians have historically realized that greater beauty allows them to attain greater status in society. Did you know the bikini has its origins in Brazil? A common saying in Brazil is "beauty opens doors." And indeed it does. But Brazilians also perceive beauty as something to which each of them is entitled and something required of them by society. Men and women both ritually trim, shave, and wax their bodies in an effort to maintain their physical attractiveness.[205] So in this regard, Brazilians do not simply see beauty as sex appeal but as a social obligation. Failure to invest in one's appearance is perceived as a transgression against their culture.

Coinciding with this perspective of beauty is the belief that physical beauty is malleable. Brazilians believe anyone can attain beauty if he or she invests energies toward this effort. Through a healthy diet, weight can be controlled. Through exercise and physical activity, physical attractiveness is enhanced. Through proper hygiene and cleanliness, one's outer beauty can be highlighted. Each Brazilian thus has both the chance to be beautiful and also to reap its associated benefits. Beauty is a key factor in Brazilian equality, and most believe the ability to be beautiful is the right of every person.[206] This differs from many other cultures and significantly influences behaviors.

The second difference in the Brazilian perspective of beauty involves its association with overall health. In Brazil, having someone comment about your skin tone, your hair, your weight, or your overall physique is as common as speaking about the weather. This includes not only compliments about how one might look but also criticism as well. Brazilians believe external beauty is a reflection of overall well-being. In other words, if someone appears unattractive for various reasons, he or she is presumed to be ill or in poor health. Inner health equates to outward appearance just as inner beauty is as important as outer beauty.[207] This holistic perspective incorporates physical attractiveness into one's overall state of health. Because of this, Brazilians feel strongly about investing in their appearance.

Brazilians realize beauty opens doors and provides opportunities to become more successful and enjoy a more attractive lifestyle. But they also perceive beauty as an inherent personal right and an obligation to themselves and society at large. They also believe how they look on the outside reflects their overall health. These beliefs push them to invest in their beauty for numerous reasons. While sexuality and having greater erotic capital play a role in influencing their behaviors, social responsibility and healthy endeavors are equally important. These well-rounded incentives are why Brazilians have been recognized throughout the world as having spectacular beauty.

What's Your Motivation for Beauty?

If sexuality is a core driver for you to desire beauty, your motivation is certainly justified. Culturally, socially, and even economically, beauty and sexual attractiveness are valued greatly. Beauty creates opportunities whether we like to admit it or not, and striving toward greater physical attractiveness is as normal as striving toward higher education or unique life experiences. Each of these allows us to attain our goals more easily and enjoy better lifestyles as a result. These things naturally motivate us, and therefore wanting to be more sexy and more beautiful makes perfect sense.

Brazilians have these same motivations underlying their desire for beauty, but they also desire physical attractiveness for other reasons. Beauty reflects good health in Brazil, and therefore pursuing physical attractiveness is a health-related behavior instead of simply a hedonistic pursuit. Likewise, Brazilians feel a sense of civic duty in pursuing beauty. This coincides with their sense of community. Instead of seeking beauty for individual reasons alone, they feel obligated to look their best for others. These motivations offer more-altruistic reasons for pursuing attractiveness.

While sexuality and an enhanced lifestyle are important to us as individuals, balancing our motivations with other positive incentives is beneficial. Perhaps you have other motivations for desiring beauty that provide similar advantages. Or perhaps adopting a Brazilian philosophy appeals to you. Either way, knowing why you desire beauty is important so you can be truthful to yourself and feel confident about your behaviors in attaining greater physical attractiveness. There is no wrong answer. From many perspectives, beauty and sexuality are important personal features offering an array of benefits to our lives. And regardless of the root of our desire, beauty does indeed reflect the level of health we enjoy.

SECTION V

We Are How We Look: The Brazilian Insight

CHAPTER 16

Brazilian Cleanliness: Health and Hygiene

We have all seen the pictures of small children in underdeveloped countries with large, sad eyes staring at us, pleading with us to help make their lives better. Dirt smudged on their faces, these children lack the basics: food, water, sanitation, and shelter. As a result they suffer not only from malnutrition but also from a variety of health disorders ranging from infections and vitamin deficiencies to dehydration. Contaminated drinking water and lack of cleanliness rank among the highest health risks in many developing nations. The solution for better health and longevity are obvious for these peoples: cleanliness leads to a better life.

Brazilians interestingly have always had a strong commitment to cleanliness throughout their history. In fact, records dating back to Pedro Cabral's original discovery of Brazil describe remarkable attention to hygiene among the natives on their arrival. The report stated the private parts of the indigenous people were so exposed, healthy, and hairless that the explorers could easily look upon them without a sense of shame.[208] Based on these accounts, the Brazilian wax seems to have predated the establishment of the nation itself! This highlights how hygiene and cleanliness are integral parts of Brazilian culture and are social expectations among Brazilians. And it showcases their belief that everyone has the right to be beautiful.

Cleanliness Is Brazilianess

With Brazil's recent economic growth, many Brazilians have naturally been traveling around the world to a greater extent. Among specific destinations, Miami has noticed a significant increase in Brazilian tourism. In an effort to attract Brazilian guests, hotels in the areas have realized some specific aspects of Brazilian culture. Cleanliness ranks among the most important factors determining whether or not Brazilians will return or recommend a hotel to a friend or family member.[209] Not uncommonly, Brazilians take two showers a day, and no matter what the socioeconomic class, maintaining a spotless home is standard. Poverty is never an excuse for poor hygiene in Brazil.

This same attitude also applies to personal hygiene. Brazilians practice healthy oral hygiene regularly after every meal. Even if lunch is eaten at a restaurant, cleaning one's teeth afterward is routinely performed by most. Clothes likewise are washed regularly. Washing after each use is standard practice, which is uncommon in many European countries. Brazilians take tremendous pride in the overall cleanliness of their bodies and their appearance. Even their dress style is best described as smart casual. Rarely will you see Brazilians appearing disheveled and unkempt.[210]

Part of the normal cultural practice for most Brazilians also involves routine care of fingernails and feet. Chiropodists, experts in the care of people's feet and hands, enjoy a steady stream of clients, as most Brazilians have regular checkups. Men as well as women take good care of themselves in this regard. Manicures and pedicures are performed on nearly as many men as women in Brazil as part of a regular hygienic practice.[211] For Brazilians, outward appearance and beauty are reflections of inner health; therefore, one who looks unkempt and unclean is presumed unhealthy. Brazilians' perspective on health and beauty is holistic, and maintaining inner as well as outer beauty through proper bodily care is imperative.

That perspective leads us to proper hair care and the infamous Brazilian wax. Despite the name, the complete removal of pubic hair through a variety of techniques has existed in many ancient cultures. Japanese and Chinese practices of ancient times have such practices well recorded.[212] Likewise, the native Indians of South America in 1500 appear to have adopted similar practices.[213] Brazilians have continued the practice and as a result have gained worldly attention for it. The popularity of the Brazilian wax has increased for a couple of reasons. One is its relation to women's control over their own sexuality, while the other involves its association with enhanced beauty (particularly in an alluring string bikini!).[214]

While the origins of this practice were perhaps primarily hygienic and appearance-related, sexual incentives play a significant role in its current popularity. From a Brazilian point of view, a Brazilian wax is a means by which respect is shown to a sexual partner. The practice demonstrates a desire to please the person with whom someone is most intimate. But at the same time, a Brazilian wax creates positive self-feelings. One feels clean, sexy, and in control of one's body, which enhances a sense of self-worth and self-confidence.[215] From this standpoint, both psychological and physical benefits are received in attaining not only greater health but also enhanced beauty.

From attention to their homes to the most intimate aspects of their bodies, Brazilians perceive cleanliness as an important part of their everyday lifestyle. Through better hygiene, they feel more healthy, more beautiful, and in greater control of their lives. This creates advantages in both mental and physical well-being, empowering them along the way. And ultimately this leads to other lifestyle practices, further enhancing youthfulness and health. Indeed, cleanliness lies at the heart of the Brazilian attitude for health, youth, and beauty.

Health, Beauty, and Cleanliness

Think about the last time you felt immaculately clean. Perhaps you had been working in the yard all day and took an extra-long shower. Or maybe you treated yourself to a full-day spa to beautify yourself. Afterward you naturally felt healthy. Cleanliness is certainly linked to healthiness by deterring germs that might cause infections, but we often fail to realize the impact cleanliness has on our mental health as well. Good hygiene is important not only for the water we drink, the food we eat, and our overall living conditions, but it is also beneficial to how we conduct our lives. This is something Brazilians have known for centuries.

No one would argue that proper hygiene reduces infections and illness, enhances physical quality of life, and allows greater longevity. But at the same time, cleanliness affects us in other positive ways. When we are clean and well-groomed, we feel more attractive and healthy. Additionally, we feel in control of our own bodies and destinies. These positive feelings spill over into other areas of our lives. For example, enhanced feelings of sexuality encourage greater feelings of intimacy in our core relationships. We also have greater mental and physical energy to handle stress and the demands of each and every day.[216]

A significant motivation for maintaining a clean and attractive appearance involves our sexuality. The sexual energy we feel when we look attractive is tangible. Ultimately, this energy is the source of life. Sexual energy is important not only for procreation but also for recreation and personal transformation. The sexier we feel, the more alive we become. If we receive positive feedback about our appearance, this motivates us even more to continue our efforts.[217] Cleanliness can thus create a cycle of positive reinforcement, making us healthier, more vibrant, and more beautiful!

To demonstrate the relationship between sexuality and enhanced self-confidence, a survey of nearly 2,500 women ranging in age from 18 to 68 was conducted. The survey examined which factors were most relevant to the decision to get a Brazilian wax. The most important factors included increased youthfulness, the presence of a sexual partner, a positive self-image, and a commitment to physical attractiveness.[218] These findings show attention to hygiene indeed correlates to greater feelings of sexuality, youthfulness, and confidence. Cleanliness offers much more than a superficial benefit to our well-being.

The law of attraction states we attract those things in which we believe through our daily actions. If we suspect things are going to go wrong, they often will. But if we adopt a positive attitude, we naturally attract positive results and circumstances into our lives. Proper hygiene and attention to our appearance are means by which we attract positive health outcomes. When we invest in cleanliness, we feel better about ourselves both inwardly and outwardly. In turn, good things come our way. We may have increased energy to exercise or to plan our diets more effectively, or we may become more socially active, gaining new friends and support.[219] Though cleanliness and hygiene appear to enhance our outwardly appearance only, the health benefits we gain within are also important. This is evident within Brazilian culture. By adopting similar practices, we too can further our efforts toward more holistic health and beauty.

CHAPTER 17

Brazil's Ancient Secret: Natural Skin Care Strategies

A shopping bag overflowing with small packages lands on the bathroom vanity counter. Immediately, the owner of the recently purchased products changes into something more comfortable so she may explore the captivating promises the products have guaranteed her. One by one she applies the products according to the instructions, and she patiently waits for the miraculous conversion of her skin and appearance. But each time, the results are far less dramatic than what was advertised. And to make matters worse, she doesn't have any idea whether these are the products best suited for her. Vulnerable to the marketing strategies of the day, she tries to discern which skin cream, moisturizer, and exfoliate will transform her into the radiant and vibrant person she wishes to be. But with each attempt, little is gained and little is learned.

While many of us are quite knowledgeable about proper skin care, misconceptions about skin care regimens and products still abound. Some of us have been victims of marketing ads dating back to our youth, during which time outward appearance was critical to our social popularity. In a 2008 survey, American women were found to spend $7 billion on cosmetics and beauty services each year![220] Sweeping promises about youthfulness and beauty lured us into trying different products. And the same trend continued as we grew older with little opportunity to gain real education about proper skin care. In fact, many women today still buy the same products they did as teenagers even though their skin has changed dramatically and their routines have changed little despite a marked increase in knowledge about skin care. In this chapter we will explore natural skin care strategies to help keep your skin youthful, healthy, and beautiful without exhausting your expense account or your efforts.

Knowing the Basics about Skin

Did you know skin is considered an organ of our bodies? In fact, it is the largest human organ, making up 15 percent of our total body weight! As a complex structure, skin provides many functions. Skin protects us from our environment. It allows us to sense touch and temperature. Our skin even participates in metabolic processes, helping maintain our bodies' chemical equilibrium. But in addition to these essential functions, skin also serves many psychological roles for us. Facial blushing can reveal our embarrassment in a certain situation. Pallor may arise if we are suddenly frightened. And differences in color, tone, and quality highlight our overall level of health in many instances.[221] These latter functions of skin are perhaps the most relevant to our discussion of youth and beauty since how we look often influences our own opinion of how attractive and healthy we are.

Our skin is composed of 7 layers in total, with the outer layers (the epidermis) consisting of 5 layers, and the inner layers (the dermis) consisting of 2 layers. The deepest layer of the dermis, called the reticular layer, contains the vital structures of our skin. These include not only hair follicles and sweat glands but also capillaries and blood vessels essential for receiving oxygen and nutrients. In contrast, the epidermis provides a series of external layers of skin cells that progressively move toward the surface as cells grow and mature. Ultimately, the outermost layer of the epidermis, which consists of dead skin cells, is lost and eventually replaced by deeper skin cells.[222] Healthy skin thus relies on a constant formation of new skin cells that demand the proper environment with all the essentials.

But what exactly are the essentials? If you listened only to cosmetic advertisements, you may be led to believe skin care essentials can be obtained only through commercial products and creams. While some skin care products are clearly advantageous, many of the basic skin care strategies involve basic health behaviors that have already been discussed. Like other cells of the body, skin cells also need adequate nutrition, hydration, protection, and restoration in order to function optimally. Therefore, attending to your health in general goes a long way in creating a glowing, healthy, and youthful-appearing skin. Without consideration of these behaviors, no skin care product can help you attain your true potential for youth and beauty.

In addition to general health measures, basic skin care involves four core strategies. These include obtaining the necessary nutrients in our diets, staying well hydrated, avoiding factors that damage skin, and applying external strategies to facilitate normal skin growth. You will notice that behaviors focusing on inner health and youthfulness are just as important as strategies involving the external care of our skin. The Brazilian perspective of holistic health and beauty naturally embraces this truth, which is a key reason the words Brazilian and beautiful have become nearly synonymous.

The Four Core Brazilian Skin Care Strategies

Working our way from the inside out, one of the most important strategies for healthy and youthful skin involves supplying skin cells with necessary nutrients. For example, skin cells require numerous vitamins for optimal function. Vitamin A is an antioxidant, preventing cellular damage but also facilitating skin cell growth. Vitamin E and vitamin C are also antioxidants, but vitamin E prevents acne while vitamin C enhances the flow of oxygen into skin cells. B complex vitamins assist with many cell processes while also strengthening collagen, improving skin tone, and reducing wrinkles. And finally, minerals such as zinc and selenium help with skin elasticity and appearance.

As discussed previously, diets rich in fruits and vegetables provide many of these vitamins and nutrients, equipping our skin with its basic requirements to stay youthful and healthy. Fruits and vegetables also provide other micronutrients such as carotenoids and retinoids, known to augment skin cell function while protecting skin cells from sun damage and metabolic by-products. In fact, many Brazilians drink carrot juice and beet juice, which are naturally high in these nutrients. Carrot juice enhances skin color and pigmentation as well, which further protects skin cells from ultraviolet damage. And beet juice is known to enhance circulation to skin tissues, providing enhanced oxygenation.[223]

Hydration is the second important strategy toward basic skin care. Cells require water to function their best. In fact, 70 percent of the entire human body is composed of water! Adequate hydration allows cells to perform metabolic functions well while also helping rid our bodies of waste, toxins, and metabolic by-products. Skin in particular requires an abundance of hydration so cells in the epidermal layers have adequate fluid. If this fails to occur, skin quickly becomes tight, wrinkled, and dull in appearance.[224]

While moisturizers can help hydrate the skin, internal hydration is equally effective while also benefitting the body in many other ways. As a general rule, one should try to drink 8 glasses of water daily, which in turn will create the full, smooth, and glowing appearance healthy skin should have.[225]

While our skin protects us from our environment to a great extent, we also should invest in protecting our skin from potentially damaging factors. Our environment can pose serious threats to the health and beauty of our skin. Dry, arid climates as well as cold environments where artificial heat is common threaten skin appearance through dehydration. The use of humidifiers as well as water mist sprays can help protect our skin in such situations and avoid premature dryness and wrinkles as a result.[226] Sun exposure is also a concern, with ultraviolet rays potentially causing skin cell DNA damage. As a result, skin cells regenerate less effectively and may develop into cancerous cells. Avoiding sun and wearing appropriate clothing (including hats) can serve to protect your skin immensely.

In addition to environmental threats, our skin is vulnerable to internal toxins. Caffeine and alcohol may cause less-than-optimal skin health by favoring dehydration. Tobacco also causes reduced skin health by depleting key nutrients, such as B complex vitamins. And many substances such as preservatives may also impart negative effects on skin cell function. These substances can trigger increased oxidative stress for skin cells, which leads to premature aging. Therefore, monitoring what we eat and breathe can go a long way in promoting better skin health.

Finally, attaining beautiful and youthful skin indeed involves proper skin care habits and behaviors. While specific skin care products will be discussed later, basic skin care involves two essential practices: cleansing and moisturizing. Each of these varies depending on which type of skin you have. Most women have combination skin consisting of oily and dry skin in different areas. Oily skin tends to have larger pores with increased sebaceous gland excretions, while dry skin is the opposite. Dry skin actually increases in prevalence as we age. Other skin types involve sensitive skin with delicate, small skin pores and sun-damaged skin, which is leathery in texture, dry, and tight.[227] Depending on which skin type you have, different techniques of skin care are required.

Proper cleansing and moisturizing for each type of skin will be addressed in more detail when skin products are discussed. However, some basics are universal. For example, frequent cleansing is never ideal, and bar soaps are notorious for drying one's skin. Cleaning twice daily with an appropriate cleanser and lukewarm water is generally preferred.[228] Likewise, weekly exfoliation is common, using scrubs with very fine grains. Interestingly, it's for this purpose that Brazilians often rub their skin with wet sand while they are lying on the beach because of sand's fine nature.[229]

As an overview, these essential strategies for natural skin care provide you with the best opportunity to have beautiful, youthful, and vibrant skin. Attending to the outer skin is only part of the solution. Taking good care of our bodies through proper nutrition, exercise, and health-related behaviors equips our skin cells with the ability to function at their best. Brazil's environment offers these quite naturally, and we can also make them a part of our youth and beauty routine. As always, youth and beauty begin from within, and skin is no exception.

CHAPTER 18

International Trendsetters: Brazilian Beauty in Fashion and Style

She didn't really want to go, but her best friend had insisted. For the last several weeks since her divorce, she was resigned to staying at home. Not having a great deal of confidence and feeling every bit her age, she thought exposing herself socially didn't sound very appealing. But with great persistence, her friend had coaxed her into a fashion makeover. Reluctantly she drove to meet her friend for an afternoon of shopping.

For the next several hours, she chose one style while her friend consistently vetoed her choices, opting for a much more youthful and flirtatious selection. Eventually her resistance wore thin, and she succumbed to peer pressure. At the end of the day, she owned three new dresses with all the appropriate accessories. And while she loved them all, she couldn't help but feel uncomfortable in her new attire. Had her daughter been wearing the clothes, it would have been fine. But she felt much too old to be wearing such hip styles.

The following weekend, her friend invited her to attend a party with her. Feeling obligated to wear her new wardrobe, she looked absolutely stunning. Even she was impressed with the way she looked. Even more surprising was how she was received throughout the evening. Several times she caught men stealing glances, and her friends seem to engage her in a more jovial way.

At first she attributed the change to her new clothes, but soon she came to realize she was the focus of change. Her new appearance had brought out a side of her that had been hidden for a long time. For the first time in years she felt like her true self. The beautiful, youthful woman inside had finally been allowed to express herself on the outside.

Brazilians have long appreciated the aesthetic appeal of fashion and style. Being of a holistic mindset, they consider how they dress to be a reflection of who they are. Fashion is thus a true form of personal expression. The style, the colors, the fabrics, and accessories chosen offer a chance for each of us to creatively express who we are. And when done well, we experience a deep congruence between our spirit, our bodies, and our minds. Through fashion we enjoy the opportunity to not only appear more beautiful and attractive to others but also to reinforce the beauty and youth we feel within.

The Culture of Brazilian Fashion

With Brazilians having such a focus on cleanliness, hygiene, beauty, and appearance, their dedication to stylish fashions should come as no surprise. In fact, the second-largest industry within Brazil today is its fashion industry.[230] But despite its domestic predominance, many of Brazil's native fashion designers had little notoriety outside the country itself. Have you ever heard of Osklen or Maria Bonita? What about Rosa Cha or H. Stern? These luxury designers of fashion apparel and jewelry are common, everyday names in Brazil, but only in recent years have they gained recognition elsewhere.[231]

Being a country of people who have a deep appreciation of beauty, Brazilians are fashion consumers who not only have highly sophisticated tastes but also are well informed. Many foreign designers have learned this fact the hard way trying to sell items that fail to meet expectations. Between a heightened level of consumer sophistication and high import tariffs, outside fashion companies have had difficulty breaking into Brazilian markets, but these are only part of the challenge. The other barriers involve the ever-increasing quality of Brazilian fashions as well as an inherent loyalty of Brazilians to support domestic brands.[232] The sense of community and social support permeating the Brazilian culture influences the fashion industry as well.

In the last few years, Brazil has enjoyed strong economic conditions while much of the world suffered economic recession. The result of this boom has been an increasing number of individuals able to afford high-quality clothing and accessories.[233] While Brazilians have always presented themselves in an attractive manner, the opportunity to express themselves more fully through style is welcomed. Not only does Brazil have several top models in the world, it also boasts some of the greatest fashions. From São Paulo Fashion Week to international fashion markets, Brazil is now recognized as one of the elite nations in the fashion world.[234]

For Brazilians, clothes represent an extension of personality. The bright colors and elaborate costumes worn during Carnival reflect this passion. The same applies to the quality and design of the clothes they wear every day. Being well-dressed demonstrates you care about others around you. Looking your best is not a selfish attempt to gain recognition from others but an act of respect. At the same time, your clothes allow you to be unique and interact with others on a more personal level. These aspects of fashion have tremendous influences on our relationships, our experiences, our behaviors, and our self-image. For Brazilians, these things feel very natural. Embracing a fashionable style that fits who you are while honoring those around you creates a healthy you and a healthy community.

The Relationship between Fashion, Health, and Youthfulness

Being able to present ourselves to others through our own unique styles and through different fashions offers many personal health advantages. Looking our best not only makes us feel good about ourselves, but it also influences how others perceive us. Both of these effects of a fashionable appearance benefit us psychologically, which in turn affects the way we behave. As it turns out, the better we feel about our beauty and appearance, the more likely we will adopt positive behaviors that further promote good health.

From an emotional standpoint, we naturally feel empowered when we dress well. Have you ever considered how many times a day we see a direct reflection of our own image? It's more than you might think. From restroom mirrors to window reflections along a busy urban street, our image provides us with frequent feedback about how we look. And for many of us, we are our biggest critics. If the way we dress meets our standard of appearance and beauty, then we naturally go through our day with a smile on our face and a spring in our step. The positive energy we receive from looking our best manifests itself in the way we feel.

While these direct reflections are quite powerful, indirect reflections of our appearance are also significant. People tend to react differently around those who are highly fashionable and sharply dressed. The halo effect is a well-documented phenomenon where people attribute other characteristics to a person based on an overriding feature. For example, a person who looks disheveled may be assumed to be lazy, uneducated, and untrustworthy. But a person neatly dressed in stylish clothes is perceived as confident, credible, and intelligent. These assumptions create powerful reflections for us through the behaviors and reactions of other people.[235] As we are treated with greater respect because of the fashions we choose to wear, we receive positive feedback from others, which in turns enhances the mental image of ourselves even more.

The positive effects of our appearance mentioned thus far affect us on a personal level, but advantages also exist on a social level. For example, our social interactions tend to be more positive when we invest in our appearance and dress. Social circles expand as people naturally want to be around others who look successful, confident, and attractive. Opportunities develop as a result that otherwise would not have been available. And chances to network with individuals arise, which can further one's success and growth.[236] Therefore, fashion offers us the chance to adopt a more healthy view of ourselves internally while also projecting a more attractive representation of who we are externally. Both strengthen our psychological and emotional well-being, which fosters healthy behaviors and perspectives as we go through each day.

The association between health and fashion is understandable based on the interaction between appearance and perception. Interestingly, the same association between our appearance and a perception of youthfulness occurs as well. As is the case with the recently divorced woman at the beginning of this chapter who felt unattractive and past her prime, fashion and style can provide us an opportunity to be young and vibrant. If we desire youthfulness, we have to look the part. A youthful appearance through stylish clothes immediately opens the door for us to behave differently.[237] In fact, dressing in a more-youthful way creates a perception and expectation about us from others. This not only pertains to our physical age but also to our mental age. Bright colors, the latest fashions, and an energetic attitude tell others we are youthful, attractive, and beautiful.

We often hear you cannot judge a book by its cover, but regardless, people often do. Fashion and style should not be disregarded when considering our health, beauty, and youthfulness. Fashion is the means by which we express ourselves and the means by which we receive feedback from others. This affects us mentally, emotionally, and sometimes physically, and it is an important aspect of health and aging. From the Brazilian perspective, dress and style are simply extensions of our own beauty and personality. Fashion is thus an extension of who we are and should be congruent with how we feel. By understanding style from this holistic perspective, we can understand the importance of attaining health, beauty, and youthfulness through fashion.

CHAPTER 19

The Brazilian Approach: Plastic Versus Nonplastic Interventions

In 2008, the documentary Smile Pinki was released and ultimately received an Oscar for the best documentary short film. Set in India, the story depicts a five-year-old girl suffering from a severe cleft lip and palate. Unable to communicate well and having a deformed appearance, Pinki was not only ostracized by the impoverished community in which she lived but was also not allowed to attend school. The documentary records how Smile Train, a nonprofit organization composed of plastic and facial reconstructive surgeons, was able to surgically repair Pinki's deformity as part of its benevolent mission. As a result of the surgery, Pinki not only gained a lifestyle typical of any other five-year-old girl but also widespread recognition throughout India. In essence, the film recorded how physical unattractiveness obstructs opportunities as well as the ability to express one's self completely. And it demonstrated how surgical interventions can heal both physical and psychological wounds.

Like India, Brazil has also had its share of poverty throughout the centuries. People in need of reparative surgery to correct birth deformities have often gone without treatment in the past. Today, with Brazil enjoying a robust growth in economic power, greater numbers of people have access to such care. But they also have greater access to cosmetic surgeries aimed at improving their overall appearance. Adhering to Brazil's perspective of holistic beauty and health, even the poorest feel they have the right to attain beauty just as they perceive health care to be a right. As a result, the rise of cosmetic surgery procedures within Brazil is rising—dramatically.

Unlike other countries, Brazil seems to have a different view of what it means to be beautiful and healthy. This philosophy affects many aspects of the culture, as we have discussed, and opinions regarding plastic surgery are also influenced by these views. Plastic surgery is not without risks, and natural efforts toward health and beauty are always preferred if the result is the same. But Brazilians believe there is a place for plastic surgery in pursuing health, youth, and beauty. Understanding the basis of these Brazilian beliefs provides us with an insight into how we too can view such surgical interventions.

Plastic Surgery in Brazil

Believe it or not, Brazil is the second-largest consumer of plastic and cosmetic surgery behind the United States. But there is one significant difference between the two countries. In Brazil, the negative stigmata associated with having plastic surgery are nonexistent. While many people, including celebrities, try to hide their surgical enhancements in America, Brazilians openly showcase their latest procedures.[238] One might expect this among friends and family in a country as social and expressive as Brazil, but individuals in the public eye also speak candidly about recent cosmetic operations. One Brazilian magazine, Plastica e Beleza (Plastic Surgery and Beauty), routinely portrays celebrities on the cover who have undergone recent procedures.[239]

The justification for this philosophy concerning plastic surgery and beauty in Brazil stems from Brazilians' holistic approach to health in part. Interestingly, psychoanalysis and plastic surgery are two health-related fields that developed together during the latter part of the twentieth century in Brazil. Both fields highlight the need to attend to all aspects of health from mental health to physical health and attractiveness. And as the nation has evolved, both fields continue to be very popular in terms of improving overall well-being. Whereas psychological treatment seeks to improve the body through the mind, plastic surgery seeks to improve the mind through the body.[240] As a result, both are seen as justifiable methods for pursuing greater health.

The health benefits related to cosmetic surgery are viewed somewhat similarly to those received by Pinki in the documentary film. Though many undergoing cosmetic surgery have no gross deformity, improvement of minor imperfections or physical enhancements have the potential to improve self-esteem. According to Ivo Pitanguy, Brazil's eminent and prestigious plastic surgeon-philosopher, plastic surgery awakens the self-esteem in each individual.[241] In other words, such procedures are not performed to attract attention from others but to improve one's self-image. This in turn allows greater confidence, esteem, and empowerment for the individual. Just as doors opened for Pinki after repair of her cleft palate, similar doors open for those who not only look more attractive but also feel more attractive.[242]

While holistic health and the pursuit of total beauty factor heavily in cosmetic surgery popularity in Brazil, other motivations also exist. As previously discussed, beauty itself offers power and prestige to everyone regardless of social class. As Brazil's middle and upper-middle classes have increased in size, the ability to afford cosmetic procedures has also increased. But even those without financial resources believe beauty is an inherent right. Brazilians believe not just in legal equality but in social equality as well. Therefore, everyone should have access to cosmetic procedures to enhance beauty just as they would other health-related procedures.[243] Today, many Brazilian clinics offer free or reduced-fee cosmetic procedures such as Botox injections, chemical peels, laser hair removal, and anticellulite treatments.[244]

While cosmetic procedures have increased in Brazil, no one is recommending everyone undergo such treatments. The underlying belief is simply that physical attractiveness offers psychological advantages and that everyone should be entitled to these benefits. Whether beauty is attained through fashion, cosmetics, exercise, or surgical treatment, this same belief persists. However, pursuing outer beauty alone is not the focus. The real pursuit involves complete and total health, of which physical attractiveness and psychological well-being are important components.

Pitfalls of Plastic Surgery

We have all seen the potential disadvantages of plastic surgery. Fish-mouthed lips from excessive procedures to plump the lips, foreheads as shiny as porcelain, and zombie-like eyes from repeated eyelid surgeries are just a few of the unfortunate outcomes for some people. The more we focus on tiny imperfections in our outward appearance, the less we see a more globalized perspective of our overall beauty. We miss the forest for the trees. And in an effort to rid ourselves of every small wrinkle, we eventually attain the exact result we were hoping to avoid.[245] Instead of creating a more youthful look, we highlight our age because of the progressively unnatural appearance we take on as the procedures accumulate.

When we live in a culture obsessed with external appearances only (at the expense of holistic beauty), we often find insecurities about attractiveness become more common. Cosmetic surgery becomes the means for a quick fix by which this insecurity can be resolved.[246] But the results are often temporary at best. Youth for many societies is glamorized to the point that everyone seeks to look as if they were still in their twenties. But youth and youthfulness are not necessarily the same thing, and youth and beauty do not always go hand in hand.[247]

Just as we must accurately define health from a holistic viewpoint, we must also define beauty in a comprehensive manner. Physical attractiveness is important, but this alone fails to define overall beauty. True beauty occurs when there is congruence between one's inner spirit and outward expression. And when we enjoy excellent health (mental, physical, and spiritual), the ability of our beauty to be witnessed by others increases. If cosmetic procedures promote this type of congruence, then health benefits undoubtedly occur. This was the case with Pinki. But when plastic surgeries seek to create an end result in alignment with some ideal image without regard to inner beauty and health, bad outcomes become more likely.

By understanding both inner and outer beauty, we can understand that youthfulness is much more than simply looking young. In many societies, people have come to equate youth with beauty and vice versa. But many people with wrinkles have greater beauty and youthfulness than thousands in their twenties. The goal is not to create a twenty-year-old, wrinkle-free appearance through surgical treatment. This alone does not create youthfulness and true beauty, nor does it necessarily facilitate long-term health.[248] The goal is to attain total health through a variety of behaviors that naturally bring about youthfulness, happiness, and attractiveness. Plastic surgery is simply one tool among many toward this goal.

Pursuing health, beauty, and youthfulness through cosmetic surgery must therefore be considered from several perspectives. Like most Brazilians, we must adopt a comprehensive view of health and beauty in order to make wise decisions about cosmetic care. Feeling more youthful and behaving more youthfully are not necessarily accomplished by eliminating sags and wrinkles. Diet, exercise, relaxation, sleep, and many other behaviors go much further in promoting longevity and well-being when compared to plastic surgery options. Only when a cosmetic procedure lets us be more fully who we are should we add this to our pursuit of health and beauty.

SECTION VI

A Prescription for Youth, Brazilian Style

CHAPTER 20

Adopting a Brazilian Attitude

In order to embrace the power of Brazilians in attaining health, youthfulness, and beauty, we must first appreciate the pervasive influence of the Brazilian attitude and culture. Through their positive energy, Brazilians naturally bring beauty and health to themselves through the law of attraction. By existing in a culture of many ethnicities, they enjoy natural diversity, which fosters greater creativity and openness. Through expression, they address life stresses as they appear while also relying on a broad network of social support. And finally, Brazilians are adept at stepping back and perceiving the larger perspective. This allows them to balance different aspects of life while still focusing on the whole.

The first prescription in attaining Brazilian health and youthfulness involves adopting an attitude similar to most Brazilians'. Certainly this may be hindered by the culture in which you live. But by understanding how the Brazilian approach to health provides the means by which health, beauty, and youth are attained, we can begin to practice these attitudes as well. Even when our environment may be antagonistic, we can change our own approach and perspective over time. In other words, positive thoughts and behaviors will eventually lead to positive habits. And these positive habits will lead us to our goal of health, beauty, and youthfulness.

The following represent steps each of us can take to adopt a Brazilian attitude toward health and youthfulness. With this in place, subsequent prescriptions involving diet, exercise, and personal care will be much easier to implement. Get ready—it's time to become Brazilian!

1. **Think Positive, Positive, Positive!**
   This is one area where science and the Brazilian lifestyle clearly agree. Thinking positive thoughts leads to positive results, especially when it comes to health. Though its mechanisms have yet to be fully elucidated, positivity is linked to healthier cells, greater capacity for cellular regeneration, and reduced disease and illness. Therefore, a positive focus not only brightens our mood but it likewise provides beneficial effects on a cellular level. This means greater health, enhanced youthfulness, and greater longevity.

   Brazilians have always adopted such a perspective. Even when times have been tough, Brazilians' resilience and their dedication to look for the light at the end of the tunnel allow them to persevere. To a great extent, this positivity comes from faith and hope that their efforts will eventually be rewarded. By all accounts, Brazilians are not ones to nag or focus on the negative. Likewise, they don't sweat the small stuff. Through spiritual strength, mental determination, and a positive outlook, Brazilians are proven survivors. They attract good things, including good health, as a result. Adopting a similar outlook on life can likewise benefit us. Bring hope, faith, and positivity into your life, and you will enjoy greater feelings of youthfulness as well as greater overall health.

2. Don't Be an Island

Being independent has advantages. For example, being autonomous puts us in charge of making our own decisions. We become self-sufficient. We are free to pursue whatever goals we wish without anyone else's input. But being solo also has disadvantages. Without a broad social network of close friends and family members, we often lack resources for support when we become overwhelmed, stressed, or burdened. We are forced to take on all the stress ourselves and hold ourselves alone accountable for whatever happens. If stress becomes excessive, our health suffers. And chronic stress leads to changes that accelerate the aging process.

Brazilian culture is unlike societies where independence and autonomy are held in high regard. Instead, community, family, and friendship are honored above the individual. Because of this, social networks are strong, offering powerful support in times of need. And while this alone provides a tremendous advantage for health and well-being, this attitude also shifts responsibility away from the individual and onto the collective. Less pressure is placed upon a single person as a result. In short, better social support equals less pressure, less stress, and a greater sense of belonging. These aspects aid our mental well-being, and in turn we enjoy better physical health as well. Greater longevity, fewer stress-related wrinkles, and a lighter attitude naturally follow when we have a number of people we can lean on for support.

3. **Embrace Diversity**
   Globalization has introduced the world to diverse ideas, cultures, and behaviors, and some interesting outcomes are occurring as a result. Diversity offers us the chance to expand our views of what is possible in life. When embraced, diversity teaches openness and fosters creativity. Through it we learn new ways to achieve health, beauty, and youthfulness while inviting positive energies into our lives. However, when we resist diversity, we resist change and become close-minded. Negative thoughts arise, inviting prejudices, biases, and false assumptions. As a result, we fail to reach our true potential as our social networks become constrained and our outlook on life becomes increasingly negative.

   Brazil, on the other hand, has become well adapted to diverse populations. Throughout their history, Brazilians have realized that diversity offers greater opportunities for innovation and creative thinking. Diversity offers also both social expansion as well as personal growth. No longer are problems seen as unsolvable. Diversity teaches that more than one solution may exist, and creative efforts will ultimately lead one to the right solution. It also teaches acceptance of others, which further fosters positive emotions and feelings. As discussed, all of these seemingly intangible factors have very tangible effects on our well-being. And openness and creativity are natural characteristics of youthfulness. Embracing diversity thus gives us an attitude well aligned with achieving better health.

4. **Express Yourself**

   Brazilians are expressive people. If they have problems, they let others know about them. If they have opinions, they share them. While Brazilians are courteous and respectful of others and avoid conflict when possible, they openly express their uniqueness. As a result, emotions are not locked inside, creating the potential for negative effects later. Social relationships are more open and understanding as a result of better mutual understanding. And social skills leading to broader support develop over time. All of these benefit health and youthfulness over time.

   Verbal expression is only one way Brazilians express themselves. Personal expressions are also seen through dance, fashion, cuisine, and even body language. This alludes to their holistic perspective of health in general and allows them easily to link health, beauty, and youthfulness together as one. Therefore, the adoption of a Brazilian attitude involves not only better verbal expression but also a more congruent expression of who you are in all aspects of your life. These representations will empower you, make you feel more invigorated, and create positive energies for you both inside and out.

5. **Insist on Balance**

   Within our bodies, equilibrium and balance among many physiological processes are essential for life. This is called homeostasis when referring to the human body. But the same concept is important regarding the way we live. In other words, a better-balanced lifestyle fosters better homeostasis and health for our bodies.

For example, working too hard without adequate "down time" often creates stress, anxiety, and negative emotions. Being overly active mentally or physically, without adequate sleep and rest, often leads to illness. In order to best promote optimal health, insisting on a balanced lifestyle is important.

A balanced lifestyle is well understood in Brazil. Despite an intense work ethic, Brazilians make time to relax, socialize, and celebrate on a regular basis. Some communities in Brazil still insist on siestas as part of their daily routine. Because of this, their bodies and minds remain fresh and restored. They maintain equilibrium and balance. And as a result, they often enjoy better health from every perspective. With better health comes greater energy, vibrancy, and youthfulness. Insist on balance within your life, and you too will reap these same benefits of well-being.

6. **See the Holistic Picture**

    Most importantly, envisioning health, beauty, and youthfulness from a holistic perspective portrays the core Brazilian philosophy regarding well-being. Beauty is not defined by physical attractiveness only but instead represents both inner and outer beauty. Likewise, our external appearance is a reflection of our inner mental and physical well-being. Dissecting the body and mind into organ systems, organs, or even cells is important to gain a deeper scientific understanding of health and aging, but ultimately all are interrelated. Brazilians understand this clearly, which is why beauty is such an important aspect of their culture. Health, youthfulness, and beauty are simply different components of a whole.

With a holistic perspective, we can see that looking young on the outside does not necessarily equate to beauty or health. We can also see the importance of investing in one's appearance since this has effects on our psychological well-being. Once we come to this realization, we can let go of the many stigmata that surround beautification and the pursuit of youthfulness. By appreciating each of these holistically, we can pursue total health while also focusing on these specific areas. The ultimate goal is holistic health, and if attained, beauty and youthfulness fall naturally into place.

7. **Have a Cafezinho!**
When business deals are conducted in Brazil, one of the traditions when dealings are positive involves having a cafezinho. This espresso-size coffee represents much more than a simple drink. Instead, it also symbolizes a level of friendship and mutual respect among the Brazilians when socializing, meeting someone new, and during business meetings. Like a handshake and a kiss on the cheek, a cafezinho is a way to endear someone and call him or her your friend. Such a tradition is important to Brazilian culture, and in fact refusing a cafezinho can be interpreted as rude or as a rejection.

Though having a cafezinho is customary in many relations in Brazil, the philosophy behind having a cafezinho with a colleague or friend demonstrates an important aspect of Brazilian culture. Like their perspective of health, everything in life is seen as connected. Therefore, friendship and business deals can mutually exist and should exist from their perspective. Likewise, the tradition demonstrates how relaxation and taking a moment to enjoy another's company is valued. Life's too short to stress over silly details or worry about what might happen. Instead, take time to see the world around you and meet those who cross your path. Having a cafezinho break is simply a Brazilian metaphor for life: appreciating everything around you and accepting everything will turn out as planned.

Brazilian culture has fostered the above perspectives on health, beauty, and youthfulness through its unique heritage, lifestyles, and environments. Adopting a Brazilian-like attitude may be challenging in other cultures or societies, but we can still appreciate why these perspectives have such benefits on our overall well-being. Though the right attitude is only one part of the overall prescription in pursuing greater health and wellness, it does serve as a foundation. With the right attitude, embracing the other recommendations for health, beauty, and youthfulness will be as easy as Brazilian tropical fruit pie!

CHAPTER 21

Youth-Promoting Brazilian Recipes

It's no secret Brazilian food can be quite a treat. The wide variety of foods native to Brazil offers a broad range of tastes and delicacies. But like any cuisine, some food choices are healthier than others. And often, healthy meals can be a challenge in not only locating the necessary ingredients and having time to prepare them but also on the pocketbook. Having wild salmon several times a month may be healthy, but budgeting for and preparing it often poses difficulties.

With this in mind, the recipes provided in this chapter are highly nutritious foods endemic to the Brazilian culture. In today's modern world, attaining these foods is much easier than in decades past, but even still, many may be hard to locate or be somewhat pricey. If you are fortunate enough to have access to these foods, their nutritious value in promoting health and slowing the aging process is tremendous. As a result, making these foods part of your dietary routine offers great benefits. But if they are inaccessible, some basic rules of thumb can be used in selecting a diet prone to enhancing youth, health, and beauty.

The first rule of thumb is natural and organic foods offer the highest nutritional value while avoiding potentially harmful chemicals, preservatives, and other toxins. While such foods may be more costly at the grocery store, farmers' markets offer great alternatives pricewise. These foods, coming from smaller farms, are typically fresh as well as affordable. Though not always the case, such fruits and vegetables are also less likely to be cultivated with foreign chemicals or other artificial processes.

The second rule of thumb is that raw, fresh vegetables and fruits provide the greatest amount of healthy nutrients. When vegetables or fruits are cooked, some of their nutritional value is often lost. Vitamins, minerals, and other micronutrients are composed of structures that can be damaged by heat or extreme temperatures. But if they are eaten in their natural state, they provide wonderful sources of nutrition for our bodies. This, combined with the fact that some types of cooking such as roasting and grilling create age-accelerating substances (AGEs), should encourage us to eat plenty of raw and natural foods.

The third rule of healthy eating involves the types of carbohydrates and sugars we choose to eat. As previously discussed, refined sugars and easily digested carbohydrates accelerate aging. With rapid increases of glucose in the bloodstream, age-accelerating glycosylation becomes more prevalent. Also, the conversion of glucose to fat and the development of insulin resistance become more likely. Whenever possible, we should choose to replace processed sugars with natural sugars to help avoid these problems. Natural sugars, unlike processed sugars, are usually packaged naturally with high amounts of dietary fiber and other nutrients. This not only slows absorption, preventing a rapid rise in blood sugar, but it also provides important youth-promoting nutrients simultaneously. Sweeten foods with honey or some other natural alternative instead of sugar when possible. Choose fruits for desserts instead of processed, sugary sweets. These choices will help you become healthier as well as more youthful.

Finally, variety is the spice of life. Just as Brazilians appreciate a balanced life between work and play, dietary variety offers a similar balance. Science has much to learn about the numerous types of micronutrients in the hundreds of natural foods available to us, and even less is known about how each benefits our bodies. But we don't need to wait for science to catch up with nature. Instead, choose a variety of healthy foods to ensure you receive a full complement of nutrients needed. With this in mind, here are a variety of recipes containing powerfully nutritious Brazilian foods that offer great potential toward our goals of health, beauty, and youthfulness.

Açaí Berry Cereal Treat (Breakfast)

Servings: 1
Ingredients: 1 cup açaí berry pulp
              Slices of fresh fruits of your choice
              1/2 cup skim or soy milk
              1 sliced banana
              1/2 cup cereal flakes

Directions: Mix açaí berry pulp, milk, and sliced banana in a blender. Place in a bowl and put cereal flakes and fresh fruit slices on top. Enjoy!

Estimated Calories: 350
Key Nutrients: vitamin A, vitamin C, iron, calcium, flavonoids, anthocyanins, dietary fiber

Brazil Nut Clusters (Snack)

Servings: 20 clusters

Ingredients: 1/2 cup sliced Brazil nuts
1/4 cup sunflower seeds
1/2 cup chopped mixed dried tropical fruit of your choice
1/4 cup shredded coconut
1 cup oat flakes
1/4 cup honey
1/4 cup light brown sugar
1 tablespoon canola oil
1/2 teaspoon vanilla
1/8 teaspoon salt

Directions: Mix oats, Brazil nuts, and sunflower seeds in a bowl thoroughly and then spread on baking sheet in a single layer. Bake at 350°F in the oven for 13-15 minutes. Place in a bowl and stir in tropical fruit and shredded coconut.

In a saucepan, heat honey, sugar, oil, vanilla, and salt over low to medium heat. Once melted, stir into oat, nut, and fruit mixture. Place mixture in a square metal baking pan lined with parchment paper and heat at 300°F oven for approximately 25-30 minutes. Let cool for 15 minutes. Break into small clusters.

Estimated Calories: 250 for four ounces
Key Nutrients: vitamin E, B complex vitamins, selenium, iron, calcium, dietary fiber

Cupuaçu Milkshake (Dessert or Snack)

Servings: 2 milkshakes

Ingredients: 1 cup cupuaçu pulp
2 tablespoons chopped lemongrass
2 cups skim milk
2 tablespoons honey

Directions: Place lemongrass, milk, and sugar in a blender and mix for 1 minute. Then transfer mixture to a container with the use of a strainer. Let the mixture freeze for approximately 20 minutes.

Pour half of the cupuaçu pulp into each of two large glasses. Then spoon the lemongrass mixture from the freezer onto both. Enjoy!

Estimated Calories: 175 per serving
Key Nutrients: vitamin D, calcium, flavonoids, quercetin

Chayote Squash (Lunch or Dinner Side Item)

Servings: 2

Ingredients: 1 chayote squash cut into strips
1 tablespoon olive oil
1 minced clove of garlic
1/2 teaspoon salt
1/2 teaspoon white sugar
1 tablespoon red wine vinegar

Directions: Heat olive oil in saucepan over medium heat. When oil is hot, add garlic, squash, salt, and sugar. Mix thoroughly and allow to cook for approximately 3 minutes.

Add red wine vinegar to the mixture and allow to cook another 2 minutes until the squash is slightly wilted but still firm. Season with additional salt and pepper to preferred taste.

Estimated Calories: 80 per serving
Key Nutrients: vitamin C, vitamin B6, vitamin K, folate, manganese, copper, magnesium

Acerola Red Sauce (Use as tomato-like sauce)

Servings: 10

Ingredients: 1 pound acerola
1 quart water
1/4 cup chopped parsley
1/8 teaspoon salt
1/8 teaspoon pepper

Directions: In a heavy saucepan, bring acerola with two quarts cold water to a boil using medium to high heat. Allow to boil for 5 minutes. Remove acerola, drain, and allow to cool slightly for 2-3 minutes. Then blend completely in a blender.

After blending, pass the resulting acerola pulp through a fine sieve and place in a medium saucepan. Add parsley, salt, and pepper as well as any other red pasta sauce seasonings you like. Bring to a boil over medium heat and allow to cook for 10 minutes, stirring occasionally. Once thickened, sauce is ready.

Estimated Calories: 30 per serving
Key Nutrients: vitamin C, vitamin A, carotenoids, flavonoids

Maracuja Mousse (Dessert)

Servings: 6

Ingredients: 8 passion fruits or frozen pulp equivalent
1 tablespoon white sugar
14 ounces condensed milk
2 cups light cream

Directions: Break passion fruits into halves and empty contents into a bowl. Rinse juice out of the skins with a small amount of water. Soften pulp manually and then strain through a fine sieve. Stir sugar and condensed milk into the pulp.

In a chilled bowl, beat cream until stiff. Place 1/3 of the cream into the passion fruit mixture. Then quickly fold the remaining cream into the bowl until no streaks remain. Refrigerate for 1 hour.

Estimated Calories: 135 per serving
Key Nutrients: vitamin C, niacin, potassium, beta-carotene, lycopene

These native Amazonian and Brazilian foods have provided a vast array of nutrients for the inhabitants of Brazil for centuries. Diet is without question part of the reason youthfulness, health, and beauty are common to the Brazilian people. Of course, having such foods does not always mean wise dietary choices are made, nor does it imply similar benefits cannot be obtained from other varieties of fruits and vegetables. If these nutritious Brazilian foods are available to you, adding them to your dietary regimen will undoubtedly be beneficial. But if not, adopt the basic rules of healthy dieting outlined to guide your eating habits. As a result, you too will reap the benefits.

CHAPTER 22

Brazilian Passion for Fitness

For some people, the words fitness and exercise do not necessarily bring to mind fun-loving images. You may have enjoyed moments of exhilarating fun and excitement at times, but at some point, incorporating a fitness routine into your busy schedule became drudgery. For example, the first time you signed up at the health center, the newness of the step machines and social environment offered some excitement and novelty. But weeks later, as the newness wore off, the monotony of a routine slowly took its toll on your level of commitment. The next thing you knew, you were paying for a gym membership you rarely used.

Life wasn't meant to be so boring or laborious! Life as well as fitness should be fun, enjoyable, and something to which we look forward. But if that's the case, what's been missing? Passion. In examining Brazilian culture, we see how passion permeates so much of its people's lifestyle. Celebrations, work, and exercise are all approached with a sense of excitement and wonder. Their positive attitude and ability to include others in their lives is a big reason why their passion is so prevalent. In order for us to make fitness a regular and enjoyable part of our health routine, we too must infuse a sense of passion into what we do.

With this in mind, the following prescriptions are some steps by which we can attain a more fulfilling and satisfying exercise routine. By adopting a Brazilian attitude about health and fitness, we too can find passion in our pursuits. And while we envisioned fitness achieving some specific goals, we soon find the benefits are far more extensive than we could have imagined.

1. **First of All, Have Fun!**
   Why do you think going to the gym was so exciting your first visit? Because it was fun! You were around new people and an active environment. You probably had on an iPod and were listening to your favorite music. Each new exercise machine was fascinating and intriguing, offering the promise of being in better shape. But after a few visits, the fun evaporated because the newness wore off. Likewise, the activities soon became less social and without immediate excitement. In time, the lack of fun meant a lack of enthusiasm, and this eventually meant a lack of commitment.

   The first step to adopting a healthier fitness routine is to make exercise fun again. People define fun differently, so only you know what raises your excitement level and enjoyment factor. Perhaps fitness with a group is attractive because you find socializing fun and it allows you to be distracted from the more unpleasant aspects of exercising. Maybe activities with immediate feedback suit your needs. Basketball, soccer, and other team sports can meet both of these criteria. Possibly incorporating dance and music with exercise creates a more pleasant environment. These are all characteristics employed by many Brazilians in their fitness routines. Find the fun in your routine, and you will soon find passion.

We naturally look forward to fun activities. Today, many options for enhancing fitness with fun are available. Meet-up groups, civic organizations, community sports leagues, and activities clubs are numerous. And if you can't find one you like, start your own! Making sure your exercise routine is fun is your first priority.

2. **Mix It Up**

   Any activity can become mundane and boring if we do it too often. This can be particularly true regarding exercise. A certain level of inertia exists, which we often must overcome in order to meet our fitness goals. While the fun meter increases our ability to do so, monotony works in the opposite direction. Therefore, it is important we constantly mix up our fitness routines to avoid struggling with this obstacle. Brazilians achieve variety by ensuring their lives are balanced. Work is balanced with play, activity is balanced with relaxation, and social interactions are balanced among many relationships. By the same token we should balance our exercise activities with a variety of different things we enjoy.

   Just as different foods offer different nutrition, different types of activities provide different benefits to our health. The theory behind cross-training is based on this simple truth. For example, it's not uncommon for a person to initially lose weight by performing a certain exercise such as jogging, only to stagnate later on. The treadmill may still tell you 300 calories are being burned, but your body no longer appears to be reacting in the same manner. What happened? Your body essentially became more efficient in performing the task. With cross-training, we continually shock our bodies, preventing them from ever getting too comfortable with one specific routine. As a result, the health benefits continue while we get to enjoy different types of exercise. Variety is a great way to help ensure our passion for fitness remains high.

3. **Rethink Your Goals and Rewards**

   What's your main goal when you start an exercise program? Is it to lose weight? Become more tone? Improve your shape? Look more youthful? All of these are excellent goals, but unfortunately, seeing tangible results can often be delayed. If we rely on tangible change as our main reward for exercising, then we may lose interest when we fail to realize results quickly enough. In order to maintain your passion and keep fitness fun, you may need to rethink these rewards. In doing so, this sometimes requires a shift in how you think about exercise and fitness.

   Like Brazilian holistic philosophy, fitness should be a part of our daily regimen to become healthier in total. While goals such as weight loss and achieving a better figure are fine, our real focus should be on achieving better total health. If we strive for healthier ways of living in all areas of our lives, everything else will naturally follow. We will eventually achieve our ideal weights while also experiencing better mental and psychological health. And we will naturally look more youthful and vibrant.

   Secondly, some rewards for exercising should be immediate. Scoring a goal during a soccer game, meeting new people at a fitness group, or running a longer distance than the day before might be some examples of instant rewards. And if we align these instant rewards with what we enjoy the most, exercising becomes self-motivating. Only you can determine which rewards provide value to you and which don't. But identifying short-term prizes that offer continued incentives to exercise will be a definite win-win.

4. **Seek Positive Feedback**

    Redefining rewards is a great way to restructure personal feedback for our efforts. But we can also enhance our passion for fitness activities by seeking a broader range of support. This is natural for Brazilians for two reasons. First, they enjoy large social circles of family members, friends, and acquaintances with whom support can be gained. And secondly, they have no issues asking for support or commenting about someone's physical attributes (positively or negatively!). For example, when Brazilians join soccer leagues, they make sure everyone is aware of their pursuits. And if they should happen to score a goal, they will really have a story to tell!

    By sharing our fitness efforts with others, we allow others to encourage and support us. And when we likewise support friends and family members in their activities, we invite them to mutually support us as well. In contrast, when we internalize our goals and activities, we rely solely on our own encouragement. While this may be enough for some people, many of us could benefit from a wider circle of support. When we let others in on our motivations, goals, and activities, we open the door for others to fuel our own passion for pursuing a healthy and more youthful lifestyle.

5. **Treat Yourself Well**

    Pursuing health and youthfulness is best viewed as the pursuit of a balanced life. Fitness and exercise are important parts of attaining health goals, but sacrificing other important aspects of health to exercise can be detrimental. For instance, burning the candle at both ends in order to make time for a fitness activity can have negative effects due to lack of rest. The body, particularly when exercising regularly, needs adequate sleep and relaxation in order to restore itself. Likewise, exercising at the expense of other important priorities can lead to increased stress. This also can trigger negative health effects.

    Learning from the Brazilian perspective of a balanced lifestyle teaches us to treat ourselves well. Prioritize those things most important to you, and then allocate time wisely in order of their importance. If heath, youthfulness, and beauty represent major goals for you, then make time for fitness as well as adequate rest. Other activities may need to be reduced or other responsibilities be forfeited. Only you know your priorities. But trying to squeeze fitness into an already packed schedule usually leads to frustrations. And this usually leads to unhealthy results in the long run.

Fitness and exercise have many health advantages for us. In addition to rejuvenating body tissues and improving circulation, fitness also reduces stress, improves sleep, enhances our immune system, and creates a positive self-image. All of these improve our total health while also promoting youthfulness and beauty. By making sure passion and fun are at the heart of our fitness routines, we can avoid many of the pitfalls often faced when trying to consistently exercise. There's a reason Brazilians enjoy being physically fit and in shape—it's because exercise is simply one more way in which they express their passion for healthy living and persistent youth. There's no reason we cannot enjoy the same thing in our lives as well!

CHAPTER 23

Skin Products with Some of Brazil's Best-Kept Secrets

Skin types are as diverse as people are. Some have sensitive skin, while others have oily skin. Some people tan easily due to an abundance of melanin-producing skin cells, whereas others are quite fair. Knowing which type of skin type you have is important because this allows you to properly care for your skin. The first step in protecting your skin and helping promote beauty and youthfulness is natural skin care as already discussed. Attention to diet and nutrition, hydration, and protection from the sun are essential. But in addition, proper cleansing, moisturizing, and exfoliation are similarly important. Knowledge about skin care products can thus be very helpful in deciding how best to care for your skin.

Brazilians value the health of their skin just as they value other aspects of their appearance and health. Healthy-appearing skin implies one is healthy within, and glowing skin naturally imparts a perception of youthfulness and beauty. Brazilians have a diet rich in foods that offer advantages to skin health. Many native fruits and plants offer tremendous benefits. From aloe vera to papaya leaf extract, Brazilians enjoy an environment conducive to healthy and youthful skin. In this chapter we will explore some of these substances native to the Amazon while also discussing other beneficial products that aid in proper skin care.

Skin Cleansing

As we go through our daily activities, we naturally accumulate microscopic debris on our skin. From dust to grime, makeup, and sweat, small, particulate matter can build up on the skin surface and potentially clog pores, cause acne, and diminish our skin's appearance. Cleansing therefore becomes an important daily activity in our efforts to maintain healthy and youthful skin. Failing to clean our skin safely and effectively can lead to premature wrinkles and aging as well as an unhealthy appearance. But while cleansing is important, it must not be performed too often. Knowing your skin type and the right skin care cleanser is the first step in pursuing youthful, beautiful skin.

In general, bar soaps should not be used to cleanse facial skin. Particularly with dry and sensitive skin types, soap can deplete the skin surface of oils needed to moisturize and hydrate cells. Soap can leave skin looking dry, cracked, and unhealthy. Instead, cleansing gels or creams are preferred. Depending whether you have dry, sensitive, normal, or oily skin, cleansing creams combine oils, wax, and water in different proportions to meet your needs. And while everyone should cleanse his or her skin once daily, those with oily skin or increased exposure to dust and debris should cleanse as often as twice or three times daily.

Skin Exfoliation

As previously described, the skin has seven different cell layers, including the outer layers that continually shed dead skin cells. This ongoing process is the reason exfoliating your skin on a regular basis is important. Dead skin cells cause both cosmetic and health-related problems when they hang around on the skin's surface too long. They can clog up skin pores, increasing the risk of acne while also interfering with cosmetic applications. Ultimately, they dull your skin's appearance and cause you to look less youthful than you should. But by ridding the skin surface of this excess baggage, better skin health is quickly achieved.

The best time to perform skin exfoliation is in the morning. Through the night, skin cells regenerate in the lower layers of skin, causing the outer layers of dead skin cells to increase. Therefore, exfoliation every morning allows your skin to be refreshed and appear more vibrant and healthy. With dead skin cells removed, cosmetic foundations can also be applied more evenly for better results. Likewise, moisturizers subsequently applied are able to reach viable skin cells for optimal effect.

While a soft washcloth in lukewarm water can serve as a gentle exfoliate, using skin care products can produce better results. This is particularly true for oily and dry skin types. Some chemical exfoliates use mild acids that gently remove debris from the skin by breaking keratin bonds or by aiding digestion of dead skin cells. Those with sensitive skin, however, may want to avoid acid exfoliates if they trigger irritation. In addition to acids, retinoids enhance skin cell turnover, facilitating exfoliation at a faster pace. Regardless which exfoliate you choose, the key is to perform the routine daily. In doing so, you give your skin the best chance for health, youthfulness, and beauty.

Skin Moisturizing

All skin types need some degree of moisturizing. While some think oily skin is already moist enough, even this skin type requires moisturizing. Moisturizers provide several benefits to skin besides hydration. They protect sensitive skin from irritants while also improving skin tone and texture. Even skin color improves and imperfections are minimized when skin is well hydrated and moisturized. Moisturizers should be applied after cleansing and exfoliation for two reasons. First, cleansing and exfoliates can dry skin, which can be reversed with moisturizer applications. Secondly, after dirt and debris have been effectively removed from the skin surface, moisturizers offer their greatest benefits by having better access to healthy skin cells.

Choosing a moisturizer depends on your skin type. Oily and normal skin types have the best results with water-based moisturizers that have light oils, while dry and mature skin types benefit more from heavier, oil-based products. Sensitive skin types should consider moisturizers that also have soothing ingredients. Within these general guidelines, many options of skin moisturizing products exist. Experimentation may be required to find the best product for you, but the key is to make sure you moisturize daily.

Skin Care Product Ingredients You Should Know

The scope of this chapter does not allow a comprehensive discussion about every cleansing agent, exfoliate, and moisturizer available; however, providing an overview of some of the more common ingredients in skin care products can be provided. Plus, some of these ingredients listed are common to Brazil and offer insights into how Brazilians have acquired an international reputation for youthful and beautiful skin.

Aloe Vera: Extracted from the aloe vera plant, this ingredient provides many benefits to our skin. As an astringent, aloe vera tightens and tones skin while also soothing damaged skin and protecting it from environmental harm. By improving circulation and promoting skin cell regeneration, Aloe also keeps skin looking fresh and vibrant. It even has some mild antibiotic and anti-inflammatory properties. Aloe is often found in many moisturizer products and is especially beneficial for sensitive, dry, and mature skin types.

Chamomile: When you think of chamomile, think soothing. Its anti-inflammatory and antiseptic properties make this ingredient ideal for skin irritated by dryness, acne, chemicals, and allergies. Chamomile also improves skin tone and reduces itching. No matter what skin type, this ingredient can be helpful in neutralizing skin irritations.

Ginseng Root Extract: While ginseng has many medicinal qualities, benefits to the skin are among its most significant. Ginsenosides are the active component of this root extract, stimulating epidermal cells and promoting cell oxygenation and rejuvenation. This gives skin a better color and appearance while also diminishing wrinkles and healing dry skin. Ginseng is present in many skin moisturizers and can be beneficial for all skin types.

Green Tea Extract: Predominantly anti-inflammatory in nature, green tea extract contains catechin and polyphenols, which protect skin from oxidative stress by neutralizing free radicals. In addition to these antioxidant and antiaging properties, green tea extract also has antibacterial benefits. This ingredient may be in moisturizers or skin protective creams and is beneficial for all skin types.

Papaya Leaf Extract: Native to Brazil and other tropical areas, papayas offer many health advantages. Specifically for the skin, it is a great nonabrasive exfoliate. Papain, the fruit's active component, is an enzyme that removes dead skin cells and impurities from the skin by facilitating cellular digestion. Papaya leaf extract reduces aging by fading skin discolorations while speeding healing of sun-damaged areas or blemishes related to acne. Papaya leaf extract is beneficial to all skin types.

Salicylic Acid: Derived from the bark of sweet birch or wintergreens, salicylic acid works as an exfoliate by breaking down keratin structures in the outer skin layers. Also known as beta hydroxy acid, or BHA, it is an oil-based exfoliate that facilitates removal of dead skin cells and other debris. It works well especially within deep skin pores, leaving the skin surface clean and rejuvenated. Salicylic acid is excellent at reducing wrinkles and helping repair sun-damaged skin. As a general precaution, however, salicylic acid may be poorly tolerated in individuals with highly sensitive skin or excessively dry skin. In this situation, water-based alpha hydroxy acid, or AHA, may be an alternative for skin exfoliation.

Ascorbyl Phosphate and Citric Acid: Derived from various fruits, these vitamin C–containing ingredients offer strong antioxidant properties. As a result, vitamin C fades skin discolorations while also improving skin tone. Its astringent properties are derived from its ability to stimulate collagen regeneration, allowing skin to tighten and reduce wrinkles in the process. Vitamin C can be used by individuals with any skin type.

Vitamin E: Also known as tocopherol, vitamin E has many benefits for skin care. Being oil-based, it is easily absorbed into skin by external application and has powerful antioxidant properties. This reduces oxidative stress to skin cells from various causes (including sun damage), allowing them to function optimally. Vitamin E also reduces skin blemishes and increases skin's ability to retain hydration, making it more youthful and beautiful. Finally, vitamin E provides ultraviolet protection from the sun. This ingredient is found in many moisturizers and sun-protective creams and is beneficial to all skin types.

Allantoin: As an extract of the comfrey root, this substance aids sensitive, irritated, and inflamed skin. In addition to its anti-inflammatory properties, allantoin also promotes new skin cell growth. It is therefore perfect for skin discolorations, bruises, and other marks left by acne or irritation. Allantoin can be used on all skin types.

Retinol Palmitate: This compound, once applied to the skin, is converted to vitamin A, which has numerous benefits toward achieving healthy skin. In addition to being a potent antioxidant and anti-inflammatory agent, vitamin A also provides ultraviolet protection to skin while promoting skin cell regeneration. This allows skin to have as a healthy, revitalized appearance by facilitating optimal skin cell function.

Jojoba Seed Oil: This wax ester is nearly identical to the composition of normal skin oil or sebum. As a result, jojoba seed extract works as a wonderful moisturizer. And because it is not water-based, it does not evaporate, allowing it to last for hours and hours.

Understanding the basics of good skin care and your skin type is the starting point for establishing healthy, youthful skin. Depending on your skin, some products may be helpful, while others may not be. Regardless, regular cleansing, exfoliation treatment, and moisturizing forms the basis for a healthy routine to deter aging of your skin. Using this chapter as a guide, you can tailor a more specific skin care routine for your unique type of skin. Ultimately, this will provide you the means to enjoy the most healthy and beautiful skin possible.

CHAPTER 24

Beauty Is Power: Brazil's Fountain of Youth

A young girl holding her violin case waited patiently in a waiting area filled with metal folding chairs. Her mother sat beside her, feeling great anticipation. They had an appointment with one of the world's top violin instructors. After submitting samples of the girl's music and speaking with several other expert violinists, they had finally been granted an audience with the master. After several minutes, the master finally summoned the girl into his studio.

"Good afternoon," the master said. "What will you be playing for me?"

"'The Devil's Trill Sonata,'" the girl replied in a timid voice.

"Indeed? This should be interesting," the master replied, knowing the level of difficulty of that particular solo.

The young girl positioned her violin against her chin and began to play. The piece was performed with perfection. In fact, the master was deeply moved in a way he had never before felt by the music. For the next several minutes he listened and watched in amazement. Once the girl was finished, he applauded with great excitement, which was quite uncharacteristic of him.

"I am stunned!" he said. "Which teacher have you trained with?"

"No one," the girl replied.
"Come now, you must have taken lessons from a professional."
"No sir."
"Then you must have studied formally."
"No. I am only eight years old."
"Then tell me dear girl, how did you acquire such remarkable talents?"
"I just play what I feel is right."

Brazilian Health: A Natural Approach

Like the master violinist, we have been influenced by how we perceive health, beauty, and youthfulness. Beauty is often considered a vain endeavor of trying to improve our physical appearance for self-promotional purposes. Youthfulness is confused with a younger look, which often focuses on eliminating signs of aging such as wrinkles and sags. And health itself is dissected into specific disorders and illnesses so we may target specific treatments against them. Many cultures and science itself lead us down this path. And when we come across a new and different perspective, we are amazed.

In much the same way, the Brazilian philosophy of health, beauty, and youthfulness challenges our current ways of thinking. Like the young girl, Brazilians simply do what feels right to them. Their ancestors have likewise behaved the same way. Without scientific instruction, they adopted a lifestyle that promotes youthfulness and beauty for centuries. As a result, Brazil has become known for its spectacular beauty, vibrant energy, and commitment to success. Brazilians just do what comes naturally. And what we are now realizing is that many of their cultural practices are indeed supported by scientific discoveries.

The Brazilian approach to health represents a holistic perspective, focusing on both the inner and outer aspects of well-being. Likewise, mental, physical, and spiritual well-being are not perceived as separate but instead interconnected entities. This provides the foundation of Brazilians' beliefs and the reasons behind their behaviors. Beauty is therefore just as important to one's health as a sharp mind and good circulation. Brazilians believe beauty is as much a social right as good health, and total wellness represents high functioning in every aspect of a person's life.

With this in mind, the Brazilian culture encourages a healthy lifestyle in several different ways. Among the most important is Brazil's natural environment, which provides numerous foods containing essential nutrients for our bodies. From açaí berries to Brazil nuts, a plethora of vitamins, minerals, and phytochemicals are readily available, allowing cells to function optimally. This in turn not only enhances health but also enables cells to perform better and regenerate themselves over a longer duration. As a result, these foods preserve health while keeping us looking young and beautiful.

Brazil's environment as well as its culture also encourages fitness and exercise. Brazilians have a range of activities in which they can partake. From martial arts to beach volleyball, an array of choices for physical exercise exists. The variety in the types of fitness activities and the different settings for each provide motivation to stay active. In addition, Brazil's strong culture of social interaction and expression makes such activities a means by which Brazilians strengthen relations and enjoy life. Ultimately, these factors create a passion not only for an active lifestyle but for health in general.

Last, the Brazilian perspective on holistic health encourages the pursuit of physical attractiveness and beauty without shame, guilt, or hedonistic incentives. Through proper skin care, fashion, hygiene and more, beauty is part of total health. Beauty and youthfulness are positive attributes that are valued by the Brazilian culture. But these facets are not pursued in isolation as they are in many societies. Instead, they are sought along with other aspects of health. For this reason, Brazil is an international leader in style and beautification because the focus is much deeper and more comprehensive than superficial beauty alone.

Combine these characteristics of Brazilians with their natural tendency to be positive, their strong sense of community, and their insistence on keeping balance in their lives, and it becomes easy to understand why Brazil is viewed as a nation of beauty, youth, and well-being. Though science does now support these behaviors as beneficial to overall health, Brazilians figured this out long ago without documented proof. They simply lived life in a way that felt right.

A Word about Beauty and Youthfulness

Would you think people were vain if they told you they wanted to be successful? What if they expressed a desire to be more intelligent? Most if not all societies assign great value to success and intelligence because they consider these to be positive human attributes. The same of course can be said of beauty and physical attractiveness. Beauty is valued by most everyone and is considered a beneficial asset. But when people speak about enhancing their beauty or performing certain beautification behaviors, they are sometimes perceived as conceited and narcissistic. As a result, feelings of shame or guilt may surface, causing them to second-guess their natural desires.

The problem with this way of thinking lies in the misperception of beauty. Beauty is often associated with external attractiveness only, and in many cultures a narrowly defined image of what is beautiful is adopted. The pursuit of this idealized image is in part where the problem lies. Beauty cannot be defined in such terms; it is always relative. Beauty encompasses not only physical attractiveness but also many other aspects. Sexuality is a strong component, as is personality, values, social skills, and more. When we confuse true beauty with physical attractiveness only, we direct our efforts and opinions in a limited way. Instead of attaining beauty through healthy efforts, we sometimes adopt unhealthy behaviors.

Misperceptions about youthfulness also exist. Youthfulness is not simply having features associated with being young. Ridding oneself of wrinkles through repeated cosmetic procedures in order to have smooth skin does not automatically create youthfulness or beauty. Youthfulness represents a feeling of vibrancy that affects us from the inside out. Through youth-promoting behaviors, our bodies function better and longer on a cellular level. This in turn naturally creates smoother skin and other physical features associated with youth. Psychologically we also are more youthful as we carry positive attitudes and stay mentally active. Youthfulness should therefore be considered holistically, in the same way we perceive beauty and health.

Science has taught us that certain foods, behaviors, and perspectives accelerate the aging process. Through oxidative stress, glycoslyation, and telomere shortening within cells, cells of every organ system often age more rapidly than they should. But by adjusting our diets, our attitudes, our appearances, and our lifestyles, we can significantly slow these aging processes. By pursuing holistic well-being, beauty and youth naturally follow.

Rather than focusing on a more youthful appearance or physical attractiveness alone, we should have total health as our goal. Brazilians have been practicing holistic health for centuries, and now science is finding this philosophy indeed has merit.

Since the beginning of time, mankind has been seeking a fountain of perpetual youth. From springs of water supernaturally blessed to modern-day medicines that promise to keep us young, these pursuits continue. In a similar way, we also long to be beautiful both inside and out. These are just natural, human desires. To date, a miraculous way of completely halting the aging process has not been found, but we do know we have more control over how quickly we age than we previously thought. As it turns out, adopting key strategies associated with the Brazilian culture offers many advantages to not only remain youthful but also to enhance health and beauty at the same time. For now, Brazilian culture offers us the closest thing to an actual fountain of youth. Adopting these strategies provides us the opportunity to reach our health goals while also giving us the youthful beauty we were always meant to enjoy.

AUTHOR'S NOTE

Is being beautiful an individual's right? What about the ability to feel sexy? Interestingly, these questions are hardly contemplated among Brazilians. Most Brazilians simply accept beauty as much of a personal right as good health. From fashion to eating healthy, beauty is the culmination of many factors. Likewise, youthfulness and healthiness according to Brazilians are best achieved by paying attention to many aspects of our lifestyle. Appreciating this aspect of the Brazilian culture can provide us with great insights into how to perceive beauty and also how we should consider youthfulness and health in general.

As a native Brazilian spending my first twenty-eight years in this wonderful country, I appreciate how Brazilians view beauty. At the same time, as a board-certified gynecologist in the United States, I have learned many have an entirely different perspective. One view has evolved over centuries of cultural tradition while the other is more scientifically based. Between these two viewpoints, I have come to realize neither is right or wrong. In fact, both offer important pieces of information valuable to us in our pursuit of health. But increasingly, both are pointing toward the same direction—beauty, youthfulness, and health are all intimately connected.

Many patients I see, women and men alike, shy away from

expressing their true desires to be beautiful. Beauty and youthfulness are seen as superficial, hedonistic pursuits, and therefore sharing such a desire with others may be perceived as egotistical and conceited. But beauty and youthfulness are so much more than what's on the surface. Through beauty, we are empowered. Through youthfulness, we are invigorated. These bolster our self-esteem and self-image. And regardless what others may suggest, both beauty and youthfulness are valued as much as monetary wealth in nearly every society in the world. My initial purpose for writing this book thus involves shedding the light on the fallacies and misperceptions that often surround how we define beauty and youthfulness. Being sexy, beautiful, and vibrant is something we all naturally crave. It's simply part of being human.

Secondly, my intention is to also share the Brazilian philosophy of health in combination with scientific evidence so that a more well-rounded view of both beauty and youthfulness can be understood. Brazilians perceive health from a holistic perspective, and therefore one cannot attain complete health without considering physical, mental, and spiritual well-being. Beauty most commonly falls within the category of physical well-being, as we look our best when we enjoy a totally healthy state. But at the same time, beauty affects our mental and emotional well-being. How can we segment health into different categories when everything is so intertwined? Brazilians through the centuries have embraced a holistic view of well-being where health, beauty, and youthfulness are all combined. And science is continually finding greater and greater support for this view.

What we now know through scientific endeavors is that how we live life affects how we age, how we look, and how long we live. Diets are important in providing our bodies not only with proper nutrients but also an array of substances known to combat the effects on aging on a cellular level. Exercise also has an important role in preserving health and youthfulness. In fact, exercise may be even more powerful than diet in this regard. And our social interactions, our spirituality, and our ability to express ourselves in every way affect our overall well-being. As science unravels each detail confirming these beliefs as facts, it becomes increasingly evident Brazilians have been on the right track for centuries. Highlighting these positive aspects of the Brazilian culture provides us a means by which we can envision how to adopt important changes in our lives. These changes are precisely the means by which we too can achieve greater youthfulness, health, and beauty.

As a believer in the human spirit, the right of every individual to pursue life as he or she sees appropriate is very important to me. Each of us is unique, and only we know what drives our own passions and desires. In my medical practice, I seek to continually empower my patients to wholeheartedly pursue their life goals and to be honest with themselves about their dreams. Institutions including science should not constrain what one feels to be right within his or her soul. The power of humanity ultimately resides within the individual because it is here where passion and drive originate. From women's rights to civil rights to human rights, individuals hold the power to change the world if only given a fair chance. And when such passions are allowed to thrive, the holistic pursuit of health is naturally empowered. Inner beauty meets outer beauty, energy meets vibrant youthfulness, and all aspects of health align in a positive way.

I am fortunate and humbled by the opportunities I have had in my life to understand health from more than one perspective. Perhaps my parents were among the most important people who taught me the importance of pursuing one's inner passion and how beauty and health are intimately connected. My father always insisted on following your heart. He believed this was the means to achieving your true destiny. And my mother showed me the importance of friends and family in providing the necessary support all of us need in life. Because of them, I cannot perceive health from the narrow lens of physiology only. Indeed, health is much more, as is the pursuit of beauty and youthfulness. In a significant way, my parents shared this vision with me, and I now wish to share it with you. I know they would be proud to have been able to witness their message spread to others.

The final section of the book concludes with several prescriptions helping you follow your passions while also attaining your goals of youthfulness, health, and beauty. This is my gift to you. But knowledge is an ever-expanding field, and new and exciting revelations continue to be discovered as time marches forward. I invite these discoveries along with any input and insights you may have about health and beauty yourself. Likewise, I extend a heartfelt invitation to any of you reading this book to be my friend.

Should our paths cross, I would gladly sit and enjoy a Brazilian *cafezinho break* with you. But until then, here is to good health and a long life. Saúde!

ENDNOTES

1. Frederickson, B. L. (2009). *Positivity*. New York: Crown Publishers.
2. Perricone, N. (2007). *Ageless Face, Ageless Mind*. New York: Ballantine Books.
3. Anonymous. (2004). *Let's Go: Brazil*. Cambridge, MA: St. Martin's Press.
4. Ibid.
5. Frederickson, 2009.
6. Ibid.
7. *Let's Go: Brazil*, 2004.
8. Ferland, M. (2012). "Uses of the Amazon Rainforest." http://www.ehow.com/about_5455690_uses-amazon-rainforest.html.
9. FruitandVeggiesMoreMatters.org. (2012). http://www.fruitsandveggiesmorematters.org/.
10. Ibid.
11. Ibid.
12. Ibid.
13. Bevins, V. (2011). "Brazil's Body Beautiful." *New York Times*. http://www.nytimes.com/2011/11/11/fashion/11iht-rgym11.html.
14. Gallon, V. (2010). *Premium Beauty News*. http://www.premiumbeautynews.com/en/Creativy-is-Brazil-s-main-asset,826?checklang=1.
15. Euromonitor. (2012). http://www.factbrowser.com/facts/7468/.
16. Models.com. (2012). "Money Girls." http://models.com/rankings/money/list.html?fnumber=5&lnumber=1.
17. Stefansson, H. (2005). "The Science of Ageing and Anti-Ageing." *EMBO Reports*, 6, S1, S1–3.
18. Drye, W. (2012). "Fountain of Youth —Just Wishful Thinking?" National Geographic. http://science.nationalgeographic.com/science/archaeology/fountain-of-youth/.

19 Ibid.
20 Reily, S. (2012). "What Do Boomer Women Want from Cosmetic Companies? Not What They're Selling." Vibrant Nation. http://www.mediapost.com/publications/article/169776/what-do-boomer-women-want-from-cosmetic-companies.html.
21 Kolata, G. (2006). "Live Long? Die Young? Answer Just Isn't in Genes." New York Times. http://www.nytimes.com/2006/08/31/health/31age.html?pagewanted=all&_r=0
22 Rattan, S. (2006). "Theories of biological aging: genes, proteins, and free radicals." *Free Radical Research*. 40 (12): 1230–38. http://informahealthcare.com/doi/abs/10.1080/10715760600911303.
23 Ibid.
24 Birren, J. E. & Schaie, K. W. (2006). *Handbook of the Psychology of Aging, 6th Ed*. Burlington, MA: Elsevier Academic Press.
25 Luevano-Contreras, C. & Chapman-Novakofski, K. (2010). "Dietary Advanced Glycation End Products and Aging." *Nutrients*, 2, 1247–65.
26 Ibid.
27 Ibid.
28 Birren & Schaie, 2006.
29 Diller, V. (2012). "Does Stress Cause Wrinkles and Gray Hair: Fact or Fiction?" *Psychology Today*. http://www.psychologytoday.com/blog/face-it/201203/does-stress-cause-wrinkles-and-gray-hair-fact-or-fiction.
30 Ibid.
31 Stefansson, 2005.
32 Kolata, G. (2006). "So Big and Healthy Grandpa Wouldn't Even Know You." *New York Times*. http://www.nytimes.com/2006/07/30/health/30age.html?pagewanted=all
33 Rattan, 2006.
34 Ibid.
35 Uscher, J. (2012). "Nutrients for Healthy Skin." *WebMD*. http://www.webmd.com/healthy-beauty/features/skin-nutrition.
36 Reynolds, G. (2011). "Can Exercise Keep You Young?" *New York Times*. http://well.blogs.nytimes.com/2011/03/02/can-exercise-keep-you-young/.

37 Birren & Schaie, 2006.
38 Taubes, G. (2011). "Is Sugar Toxic?" *New York Times*. http://www.nytimes.com/2011/04/17/magazine/mag-17Sugar-t.html?pagewanted=all.
39 Luevano-Contreras, C. & Chapman-Novakofski, K., 2010.
40 Knapowski, J., Wieczorowska-Tobis, K., & Witowski, J. (2002). Pathophysiology of ageing. *Journal of Physiology and Pharmacology*, 53, 135–146.
41 Yapp, R. (2010). "Brazil's obesity rate could match US by 2022." *The Telegraph*. http://www.telegraph.co.uk/news/worldnews/southamerica/brazil/8204625/Brazils-obesity-rate-could-match-US-by-2022.html.
42 Strom, S. (2011). "Local laws fighting fat under siege." *New York Times*. http://www.nytimes.com/2011/07/01/business/01obese.html?_r=1&ref=transfattyacids.
43 Mozaffarian, D., Aro, A., & Willett, W. C. (2009). "Health effects of trans-fatty acids: experimental and observational evidence." *European Journal of Clinical Nutrition*. 63 Suppl. 2, S5–21.
44 Strand, R., *What Your Doctor Doesn't Know About Nutritional Medicine May Be Killing You* (Nashville TN): Thomas Nelson; 1 edition May 15, 2007
45 Mozaffarian, D., Aro, A., & Willett, W. C., 2009.
46 Fries, W.C. (2012). "Natural Skin Care: The Skinny on Fats." *WebMD*. http://www.webmd.com/healthy-beauty/features/natural-skin-care-skinny-fats.
47 Fischer, N., Hammerschmidt, F., & Brunke, E. (1995). "Analytical Investigation of the Flavor of Cupuaçu (Theobroma gradiflorum Spreng)." *Fruit Flavors*. http://pubs.acs.org/doi/abs/10.1021/bk-1995-0596.ch002?prevSearch=cupuacu&searchHistoryKey=.
48 Attaway, J. (1993). "Citrus Juice Flavonoids with Anticarcinogenic and Antitumor Properties." *Food Phytochemicals for Cancer Prevention*. http://pubs.acs.org/doi/abs/10.1021/bk-1994-0546.ch019?prevSearch=flavonoids&searchHistoryKey=.
49 Sabatelli, J. "The Seven Oils." http://www.jsabatelli.com/seven_oils.html.
50 Rajan, L. (2011). "10 health benefits of Jackfruit." http://www.gingerchai.com/2011/07/05/10-health-benefits-of-jackfruit/.

51 Williams, J. E. (2011). "Amazing Amazonian Superfood, Aguaje." http://renegadehealth.com/blog/2011/11/25/amazing-amazonian-superfood-aguaje.
52 Kristie, K. (2010). "10 Surprising Health Benefits of Chayote." http://healthmad.com/nutrition/10-surprising-health-benefits-of-chayote/.
53 Ibid.
54 Thompson, C., et al. (2008). "Brazil nuts: an effective way to improve selenium status." *American Journal of Clinical Nutrition*, 87, 2, 379–384.
55 Mourvaki, E.; Gizzi, S.; Rossi, R.; & Rufini, S. (2005). "Passionflower Fruit—A 'New' Source of Lycopene?" *Journal of Medicinal Food*, 8, 1, 104–06.
56 Ibid.
57 Schauss, A. G., Jensen, G. S., & Wu, X. (2010). "Açai (Euterpe oleracea)." *Flavor and Health Benefits of Small Fruits*. http://pubs.acs.org/action/showCitFormats?doi=10.1021%2Fbk-2010-1035.ch013.
58 Connor, S. W. (2009). "Nutritional benefits of acerola cherries." *Helium*. http://www.helium.com/items/1043308-nutritional-benefits-of-acerola-cherries.
59 Office of Dietary Supplements. (2012). "Multivitamin/Mineral Supplements." National Institute of Health. http://ods.od.nih.gov/factsheets/MVMS-QuickFacts/.
60 Office of Dietary Supplements. (2012). "Omega 3 Fatty Acids and Health." National Institute of Health. http://ods.od.nih.gov/factsheets/Omega3FattyAcidsandHealth-HealthProfessional/.
61 Ibid.
62 Patel, J. (2008). "A Review of Potential Health Benefits of Flavonoids." *Lethbridge Undergraduate Research Journal*. 3, 2. http://www.lurj.org/article.php/vol3n2/flavonoids.xml.
63 Ibid.
64 Linus Pauling Institute. (2012). "Flavonoids." Oregon State University. http://lpi.oregonstate.edu/infocenter/phytochemicals/flavonoids/.

65 Brett, J. (2012). "What are carotenoids?" Discovery Fitness and Health. http://health.howstuffworks.com/wellness/food-nutrition/vitamin-supplements/what-are-carotenoids1.htm.
66 Ibid.
67 Ibid.
68 Ibid.
69 Brett, J. (2012). "Benefits of Vitamin E." *Discovery Health and Fitness*. http://health.howstuffworks.com/wellness/food-nutrition/vitamin-supplements/benefits-of-vitamin-e.htm.
70 Rajan, L. (2011). "10 health benefits of Jackfruit." http://www.gingerchai.com/2011/07/05/10-health-benefits-of-jackfruit/.
71 Brett, J. (2012). "Benefits of Vitamin A." Discovery Health and Fitness. http://health.howstuffworks.com/wellness/food-nutrition/vitamin-supplements/benefits-of-vitamin-a.htm.
72 Walling, E. (2009). "The Beauty of B: Why You May Need More of the Vitamin B Complex." *NaturalNews.com*. http://www.naturalnews.com/026357_vitamin_B_vitamins.html.
73 Office of Dietary Supplements. (2012). *National Institute of Health*. http://ods.od.nih.gov/factsheets/Selenium-HealthProfessional/.
74 Anonymous. (2012). "Health Facts : Health Benefits of Manganese." *TheResearchopedia*. http://www.theresearchpedia.com/health/health-benefits-of-foods/health-benefits-of-manganese.
75 PureHealthMD. (2012). "Basic Minerals: Magnesium." *Discovery Health and Fitness*. http://health.howstuffworks.com/wellness/food-nutrition/vitamin-supplements/basic-minerals3.htm.
76 Santos, F. (2008). "Sounds of Little Brazil, Bursting with Pride." *New York Times*. http://www.nytimes.com/2008/09/01/nyregion/01brazil.html.
77 Ibid.
78 Haas, E. M. (2012). "General Detoxification." *Healthy.net*. http://www.healthy.net/scr/article.aspx?Id=1558.
79 Kresser, C. (2010). "The Top 3 Dietary Causes of Obesity and Diabetes." http://chriskresser.com/the-top-3-dietary-causes-of-obesity-diabetes.

80 Ibid.
81 Office of Dietary Supplements. (2012). "Omega 3 Fatty Acids and Health." National Institute of Health. http://ods.od.nih.gov/factsheets/Omega3FattyAcidsandHealth-HealthProfessional/.
82 Kresser, 2010.
83 Calorie Count. (2012). "Calories in Açaí Berry Juice." http://caloriecount.about.com/calories-walmart-Açaí-berry-juice-i147119.
84 Kristie, K. (2010). "10 Surprising Health Benefits of Chayote." http://healthmad.com/nutrition/10-surprising-health-benefits-of-chayote/.
85 Calorie Count. (2012). "Calories in Açaí with Mango Juice." http://caloriecount.about.com/calories-bossa-nova-juice-i169231.
86 Calorie Counter. (2012). "Calories in Rice and Pinto Beans, Organic." http://caloriecount.about.com/calories-eden-foods-rice-pinto-beans-i104243.
87 Whole Living. (2012). "Quinoa Salad with Toasted Almonds." http://www.wholeliving.com/132688/quinoa-salad-toasted-almonds?center=0&gallery=136520&slide=132689.
88 Mascarelli, A. (2011). "Exercise counteracts aging effects." *Los Angeles Times*. http://articles.latimes.com/2011/sep/01/health/la-he-aging-physiology-20110901.
89 Puterman, E., et al., "The Power of Exercise: Buffering the Effect of Chronic Stress on Telomere Length." PLoS ONE, 5, 5. http://www.plosone.org/article/info%3Adoi%2F10.1371%2Fjournal.pone.0010837.
90 Davidson, L. E., et al. (2009). "Effects of exercise modality on insulin resistance and functional limitation in obese adults." *Archives of Internal Medicine*, 169, 2, 122–31.
91 Bjornebelck, A., et al. (2005). "The antidepressant effect of running is associated with increased hippocampal cell proliferation." *International Journal of Neuopsychopharmacology*, March 15, 1–12.
92 Gobeske, K. T., et al. (2009). "BMP signaling mediation effects of exercise on hippocampal neurogenesis and cognition on mice." PLoS ONE, 4, 10. http://www.plosone.org/article/info:doi%2F10.1371%2Fjournal.pone.0007506.

93 Kristal, M. (2009). "Shake your beauty: Improve your skin with exercise." *Psychology Today*, April 10. http://www.psychologytoday.com/blog/shake-your-beauty/200904/improve-your-skin-exercise.
94 Ibid.
95 Mascarelli, 2011.
96 Consulate General of Brazil. (2012). "Sports in Brazil." http://www.brazil.org.hk/ehtml/about_lon_sports.htm.
97 Henderson, S. (2005). "The rhythm of capoeira: Aerobic workout combines cultural music and dance for an effective exercise." *Ebony*, August. http://findarticles.com/p/articles/mi_m1077/is_10_60/ai_n14835515/.
98 Eisenthal, J. (2012). "Building the blend: How Brazil grew its ethanol industry." *EthanolToday.com*.
99 Science Daily. (2010). "Learning keeps brain healthy: Mental activity could stave off age-related cognitive and mental decline." March 2.
100 Ober, B. (2012). "Memory, brain, and aging: The good, the bad and the promising." *California Agriculture*, 64, 4, 74–82.
101 Daffner, K. R. (2010). "Promoting successful cognitive aging: A comprehensive review." *Journal of Alzheimer's Disease*, 19, 4, 1101–22.
102 Swan, G. E. & Carmelli, D. (1996). "Curiosity and mortality in aging adults: A 5 year follow up of the Western Collaborative Group Study." *Psychology of Aging*, 11, 3, 449–53.
103 Hughes, D. (2011). "Mentally ill have reduced life expectancy, study finds." *BBC News*.
104 Jones, J. W. (2010). "Life expectancy in mental illness." PsychCentral.
105 Hughes, 2011.
106 Daffner, 2010.
107 Frederickson, B. L. 2009. *Positivity*. New York: Crown Publishers.
108 OECD. (2012). "Work-Life balances —Better Life Index." http://www.oecdbetterlifeindex.org/; http://www.oecdbetterlifeindex.org/countries/brazil/
109 Ibid.

110 Frederickson, B. L. (2009). Positivity. New York: Crown Publishers.
111 Haupt, A. (2010). "How your personality affects your health." *US News and World Report*; http://health.usnews.com/health-news/family-health/heart/articles/2010/09/22/how-your-personality-affects-your-health
112 Ibid.
113 Ibid.
114 Ibid.
115 Pampel, F. C. (2011). "Does reading keep you thin? Leisure activities, cultural tastes and body weight in comparative perspectives." *Sociology of Health and Illness*, 34, 3   396–411.
116 Axelsson, J., et al. (2010). "Beauty sleep: Experimental study on the perceived health and attractiveness of sleep deprived people." *British Medical Journal*, 341, 6614.
117 Breus, M. (2007). *Beauty Sleep: Look young, lose weight, and feel great through better sleep*. New York: Plume Publishing.
118 Ibid.
119 Ibid.
120 Ibid.
121 Ibid.
122 Haupt, 2010.
123 Reimao, R. et al. (2000). "Siestas among Brazilian native Terena adults: A study of daytime napping." *Arq. Neuropsiquiatar.* 58, 1, 39–44.
124 Palka, L. (2006). "Cultural difference between Brazil and the United States." *Brazil Magazine*. http://org.elon.edu/brazilmagazine/2006/docs/Palka.pdf.
125 Grogan, S. (2008). *Body image: Understanding body dissatisfaction in men, women and children*. New York: Routledge.
126 Ibid.
127 ANAD. (2010). "Eating disorder statistics." National Association of Anorexia Nervosa and Associated Disorders, Inc. http://www.anad.org/get-information/about-eating-disorders/eating-disorders-statistics/.
128 Ibid.
129 ANAD, 2010.
130 Grogan, 2008.

131 ANAD, 2010.
132 Torres, J.P.M., et al. (2009). "Persistent toxic substances in the Brazilian Amazon: Contamination of man and the environment." *Journal of Brazilian Chemistry*, 20, 6.
133 Zielinski, S. (2008). "Exploring the Amazon rainforest." *Smithsonian Magazine*, January.
134 Van Slooten, J. (2010). "Thousands exposed to Shell's toxic waste in Brazil." *Radio Netherlands Worldwide*.
135 Watts, J. (2012). "Brazil's leader vetoes portions of new Amazon rainforest law." *The Guardian*, May 25.
136 Morrison, J. (2011). *Cleanse your body; Cleanse your mind*. New York: Penguin Group.
137 Watts, 2012.
138 Carrington, D. (2010). "Can Brazil become the world's first superpower?" *The Guardian*, August 5.
139 Watts, 2012.
140 Morrison, 2011.
141 Albert, H. (2010). "Airborne pollution linked to skin aging." *Journal of Investigative Dermatology*, July 23.
142 WorldHealth.net (2012). "Air pollution linked to chronic heart disease."
143 Willingham, S. B. & Ting, J. P. (2008). "NLR's and the dangers of pollution and aging." *Nature Immunology*, 9, 8, 831–33.
144 Migliore, L. & Coppede, F. (2009). "Environmental-induced oxidative stress in neurodegenerative disorders and aging." *Mutation Research/Genetic Toxicology and Environmental Mutagenesis*, 674, 1–2, 73–84.
145 Morrison, 2011.
146 Ibid.
147 Ibid.
148 Workman, D. (2008). "World's most emotional countries." *Suite101.com*. February 16. http://suite101.com/article/worlds-most-emotional-countries-a44851.
149 Stuart, D. (2012). "Intercultural communication: The Challenge of the multicultural work place." IOR. http://www.iorworld.com/intercultural-communication--the-challenge-of-the-multicultural-work-place-pages-240.php.

150 Gudykunst, W. B. (2003). *Cross-cultural and Intercultural Communication.* Thousand Oaks, CA: SAGE Publications, Inc.
151 World Health Organization. (2010). "Mental Health: Country reports and charts." http://www.who.int/mental_health/prevention/suicide/country_reports/en/.
152 Fernandez, I., et al. (2000). "Differences between culture in emotional verbal and nonverbal reaction." *Psicothema, 12,* 83–92.
153 Kato, K.; Zweig, R.; Barzilai, N.; & Altzmon, G. (2012). "Positive attitude toward life and emotional expression as personality phenotypes for centarians." *Aging, 4,* 5,259–67.
154 Masui, Y.; Gondo, Y.; Inagaki, H.; & Hirose, N. (2006). "Do personality predict longevity? Findings from Tokyo Centarian Study." *Age, 28,* 4, 353–61.
155 Cartensen, L. L., et al. (2011). "Emotional experience improves with age: Evidence based on over 10 years of experience sampling." *Psychology of Aging, 26,* 1, 21–33.
156 Kato, et al., 2012.
157 Frederickson, B. L. (2009). *Positivity.* New York: Crown Publishers.
158 Frederickson, 2009.
159 Cartensen, 2011.
160 Zablocki, E. (2004). "The mind-body-health connection." WebMD. http://www.webmd.com/healthy-beauty/features/mind-skin-health-connection.
161 American Psychiatric Association. (2012). "Stress in America: Our health at risk." http://www.apa.org/news/press/releases/stress/2011/final-2011.pdf.
162 Ibid.
163 Ibid.
164 Science Daily. (2011). "Depression and chronic stress accelerates aging." http://www.sciencedaily.com/releases/2011/11/111109093729.htm.
165 American Psychiatric Association, 2012.
166 Science Daily, 2011.
167 Stein, R. (2004). "Study first to confirm that stress speeds aging." *Washington Post,* November 30. http://www.washingtonpost.com/wp-dyn/articles/A20394-2004Nov29.html.

168 Ibid.
169 Carlo, G.; Koller, S.; Raffaelli, M.; and de Guzman, M. R. (2007). "Culture-Related strengths among Latin American families: A case study of Brazil." *Faculty Publications, Department of Child, Youth, and Family Studies,* 64.
170 Ibid.
171 American Psychiatric Association, 2012.
172 Carlo et al., 2007.
173 Ibid.
174 Russ. (2009). "How different cultures respond to conflict." *Walkabout Consulting.* March 19. http://walkaboutconsulting.com.au/2009/how-different-cultures-respond-to-conflict/.
175 Keller, K. (2012). "A few favorite Brazilian Portuguese expressions." *Dummies.com.* http://www.dummies.com/how-to/content/a-few-favorite-brazilian-portuguese-expressions.html.
176 Coelho, P. (2011). "The daisy and selfishness." *Paul Coelho's Blog,* February 10. http://paulocoelhoblog.com/2011/02/10/the-daisy-and-selfishness/.
177 Levin, J., Chatters, L. M., & Taylor, R. J. (2010). "Theory in religion, aging and health: An overview." *Journal of Religion and Health, 50,* 2, 389–406.
178 Mohandas, E. (2008). "Neurobiology of spirituality." *Mens Sana Monographs,* 6, 1. http://www.ncbi.nlm.nih.gov/pmc/articles/PMC3190564/?tool=pmcentrez.
179 Klatz, R., & Goldman, R. (2003). *The Science of Anti-Aging Medicine.* Chicago, IL: American Academy of Anti-Aging Medicine.
180 Ibid.
181 Ibid.
182 Konopack, J. F. & McAuley, E. (2012). "Efficacy-mediated effects of spirituality and physical activity on quality of life: A path analysis." *Health and Quality of Life Outcomes,* 10, 57.
183 Ibid.
184 Lawler-Row, K. A. & Elliott, J. (2009). "The role of religious activity and spirituality in the health and well-being of older adults." *Journal of Health and Psychology,* 14, 43.
185 Mohandas, 2008.

186 Ibid.
187 Dawson, A. (2007). *New Era, New Religions: Religious transformation in contemporary Brazil.* Burlington, VT: Ashgate Publishing, Ltd.
188 Morwyn. (2001). *Magic from Brazil.* St. Paul, MN: Llewellyn Publications.
189 Ibid.
190 Dawson, 2007.
191 Ibid.
192 Miles, A. K., Sledge, S., & Coppage, S. (2008). "Linking spirituality to workplace benefits: An analysis of Brazilian Candomblé." *Culture and Religion, 9*, 3, 211–32.
193 Vandenberghe, L., Prado, F. C., & deCamargo, E. A. (2012). "Spirituality and religion in psychotherapy: Views of Brazilian psychotherapists." *International Perceptions in Psychology: Research, Practice, Consultant, 1,* 2, 79-93.
194 Dawson, 2007.
195 Wood, N. (2002). *The Beauty Myth.* New York: Harper Collins.
196 Hakim, C. (2010). "Erotic capital." *European Sociological Review,* 26, 5, 499–518.
197 Wood, 2002.
198 Gottschall, J., et al. (2008). "The 'Beauty Myth' is no myth." *Human Nature,* 19, 2, 174–80.
199 Hakim, 2010.
200 Ibid.
201 Ibid.
202 Ibid.
203 Ibid.
204 Ibid.
205 Jarvin, A. (2010). "Cosmetic citizenship: Beauty, affect. And inequality in Southeastern Brazil." *Duke University Dissertations.* http://dukespace.lib.duke.edu/dspace/bitstream/handle/10161/2382/D_Jarrin_Alvaro_a_201005.pdf?sequence=1.
206 Ibid.
207 Ibid.

208 Ginway, M. E. (2004). *Brazilian Science Fiction: Cultural myths and nationhood*. Danvers, MA: Rosemont Publishing and Printing Company.
209 Wharton, S. (2012). "U.S. hoteliers learn how to wow Brazilian guests." *HotelNewsNow.com*.
210 Taylor, M. (2006). "Cleanliness is next to Brazilianess." Gringoes.com.
211 Ibid.
212 Ramsey, S.; Sweeney, C.; Fraser, M.; & Oades, G. (2009). "Pubic hair and sexuality: A review." *Journal of Sexuality and Medicine*, 6, 2102–10.
213 Ginway, 2004.
214 Meredith, D. (2011). "The last triangle: Sex, money, and the politics of pubic hair." *Owens University Master's Thesis: Cultural Studies*.
215 Aldrich, M. (2009). *How to Get the Perfect Brazilian Wax*. Bloomington, IN: Universe Publications.
216 Aldrich, 2009.
217 Herbenick, D., et al. (2010). "Pubic hair removal among women in the United States: Procedures, methods and characteristics." *Journal of Sexual Medicine, 7*, 10, 3322–30.
218 Herbenick et al., 2010.
219 Aldrich, 2009.
220 Buena, C. (2008). "Beauty tips that won't break the bank." *eHow.com*.
221 McPhee, I. (2008). "The physiology of skin." *Suite101.com*.
222 Ibid.
223 Agadoni, L. (2010). "Brazilian beauty tips." *ModernMom.com*.
224 McPhee, 2008.
225 Berg, R. (2001). *Beauty: The New Basics*. New York: Workman Publishing Group.
226 Ibid.
227 Derrick, J. (2012). "Skin care: My best tips to make your skin look younger." *About.com*.
228 Ibid.

229 Agadoni, 2010.
230 Interband. (2009). "What about Brazilian brands?" http://www.interbrand.com/Libraries/Articles/10_What_about_Brazilian_Brands_english_final2_pdf.sflb.ashx.
231 Anaya, S. (2010). "Inside Brazil's booming fashion industry." *The Business of Fashion*. http://www.businessoffashion.com/2010/08/inside-brazils-booming-fashion-industry.html.
232 Ibid.
233 Fox News Latino. (2012). "Milan who? Brazil taking over fashion world." *Fox News Latino*, January 16, 2012. http://latino.foxnews.com/latino/lifestyle/2012/01/16/milan-who-brazil-taking-over-fashion-world/.
234 Anaya, 2010.
235 Bonandes, R. (2012). "Top ten: Proven benefits of looking your best." *AskMen.com*. http://www.askmen.com/grooming/appearance/top-10-proven-benefits-of-looking-your-best.html.
236 Ibid.
237 Ibid.
238 Barchfield, J. (2012). "Brazil's poor get free beauty." *Huffington Post*, March 22, 2012. http://www.huffingtonpost.com/2012/03/22/brazils-poor-get-free-bea_n_1373639.html.
239 Ibid.
240 Edmonds, A. (2011). "A 'necessary vanity.'" *The New York Times*. August 13, 2011. http://opinionator.blogs.nytimes.com/2011/08/13/a-necessary-vanity/.
241 Ibid.
242 Ibid.
243 Ibid.
244 Barchfield, 2012.
245 Sommerfield, J. (2008). "Pursuit of youth isn't always pretty." *MSNBC*.
246 Bandach, A. L. (1988). "The dark side of plastic surgery." *The New York Times*, April 17, 1988. http://www.nytimes.com/1988/04/17/magazine/the-dark-side-of-plastic-surgery.html?pagewanted=all&src=pm.
247 Sommerfield, 2008.
248 Bandach, 1988.

INDEX

A
açaí 6, 34-35, 50, 161, 185
acerola 35, 39-40, 50-51, 164
adrenaline 15
advanced glycation end-products *see AGEs*
age accelerators 12, 15, 17
AGEs (advanced glycation end-products) 13-16, 22-23, 32, 41, 44, 49, 57, 87
alcohol 65, 135
allantoin 181
aloe vera 175, 178
Alzheimer's disease 13, 23, 87
antioxidant 6-7, 16, 31-35, 39-41, 43, 49-52, 134, 179-181
anxiety 14, 39, 74, 97, 102-103, 109, 156
ascorbyl phosphate 180, 207

B
beta-carotene 16, 34, 40-41, 165
brazil nuts 21, 33, 43, 51, 162, 185
buriti 32

C
cafezinho 157-158, 192
caffeine 135
carbohydrates 26-27, 34, 74, 160
carotenoids 32, 35, 40, 51, 134, 165
chamomile 179
chayote 32, 50, 163
cholesterol
    HDL 25, 33
    LDL 25, 33, 39
citric acid 180
cupuaçu 7, 31, 39, 163

D
depression 14, 39, 65, 81, 93, 97, 102-103, 109
detoxification 45-47, 49-52, 58, 89

E
exfoliation 136, 175-178, 180-181

F
fats
    saturated 24, 26, 33
    trans 21, 24-26, 33
    unsaturated 24-25
fiber 22-23, 26, 31-32, 34, 47-52, 160-162
    insoluble 26

flavonoids 31, 34-35, 39-40, 51, 161, 163, 165

G
genetics 12, 96
ginseng root extract 179
glucose 14-15, 22-24, 26, 44, 47, 49, 57, 74, 75, 103, 160
glycosylation 22-23, 26, 44, 47, 49, 57, 63, 74, 87, 160
green tea extract 179

H
hydration 49, 51, 133-135, 175, 177, 181

I
insulin 14, 22, 26-27, 41, 47, 49, 57, 74, 103-104, 160

J
jaca fruit 31-32, 43
jojoba seed oil 181

L
lipoprotein 25

M
maracujá 7, 34, 40
micronutrients 15, 26, 31, 38, 40, 42, 44, 50-51, 81, 134, 160-161
moisturizing 41, 135-136, 175, 177-178, 181
moriche palm fruit 32, 40

O
obesity 13-14, 23-24, 27, 81, 87, 102-103
omega-3s 16, 26, 38-39, 48
omega-6 38, 47-48

P
papaya leaf extract 179-180
passion fruit 7, 165
phytosterols 7
plastic surgery 144

Q
quinoa 51

R
radicals, free 12-13, 15-16, 25, 32, 39, 41, 48, 87, 179
retinoids 16, 134, 177
retinol palmitate 181

S
salicylic acid 180
sugar
    natural 22, 31-32, 48, 50, 160
    refined 14, 21-23, 32, 47-50, 160
supplements 35, 37-39, 41-44, 81
surgery, plastic 144-148

T
tobacco 12, 65, 86, 103, 135
tranquilo, fique 106

V
vitamin E 33, 41, 134, 162, 180-181

NOTES

ABOUT THE AUTHOR

Luciano Sztulman, MD, FACS, FACOG is the Chief of Gynecologic services at award-winning Boston University affiliate and academic hospital Roger Williams Medical Center in Providence, Rhode Island. He also maintains a private practice in Providence.

Dr. Luciano is a Diplomate of the American Board of Obstetrics and Gynecology, and a Fellow of the American College of Obstetricians and Gynecologists (FACOG) and of the American College of Surgeons (FACS).

Dr. Luciano has recently served as a judge for the 2012 Miss Brasil USA MA Pageant. Born in São Paulo, Brazil, Dr. Luciano is an internationally renowned women's advocate who has dedicated his professional life to women's health and wellness for more than thirty years.